A Promise Fulfilled

A Promise Fulfilled

One Couple's Journey Through Misdiagnosis, Breast Cancer and Advocacy

William C. Thiel
As told to Maureen Buchanan Jones

iUniverse, Inc.
New York Lincoln Shanghai

A Promise Fulfilled
One Couple's Journey Through Misdiagnosis, Breast Cancer and Advocacy

iUniverse books may be ordered through booksellers or by contacting:

iUniverse
2021 Pine Lake Road, Suite 100
Lincoln, NE 68512
www.iuniverse.com
1-800-Authors (1-800-288-4677)

The views expressed in this work are solely those of the author and do not necessarily reflect the views of the publisher, and the publisher hereby disclaims any responsibility for them.

ISBN-13: 978-0-595-40747-7 (pbk)
ISBN-13: 978-0-595-85112-6 (ebk)
ISBN-10: 0-595-40747-1 (pbk)
ISBN-10: 0-595-85112-6 (ebk)

Printed in the United States of America

Angels that Speak

for Maureen Elizabeth Thiel

If we listen, we'll hear
the chorus bells ringing.
If we look, we'll see
the angels come singing.

To be blessed as I
with the force from above,
you'll feel passion and honor,
God's glorious love.

I know my angel,
always present, so near.
Because of her strength,
I go forward, no fear.

Listen to your angel
delivered to you;
Carry her mission,
her story so true.

Acknowledgements

Many people helped me along this path. Their compassion and determination to make a difference are nothing short of heroic. I thank from the bottom of my heart, Dr. Lillie Shockney, RN, BS, MAS, Administrative Director of the Johns Hopkins Avon Foundation Breast Center in Baltimore, Maryland; the *Y-Me Breast Cancer Organization*; and the *Susan G. Komen Foundation*. They are all partners with one goal. The *Women's Forum* and TCI *Publicity*, knew that this story had to be told. They made tremendous efforts to get Maureen's story out.

Malcolm McGregor, Michael McDonald and Marcia Kohanski of the Foley Law Firm, believed in Maureen and fought for her for over six years. I thank them for their legal expertise and diligence, and I thank them for their unwavering friendship. My deepest thanks also go to Paul Lyon, Executive Director of the *Committee for Justice for All*. From the start, he was there to help. Without him, *Maureen's Mission* would not exist. He too is a friend.

Senator Jane Orie believed a change was needed. She, along with her assistant, Joanne Marino McGreevy, relentlessly worked on a legislative Resolution and Bill to end misdiagnosis and delayed diagnosis. I do not have enough words for what that means to me. Thank you, Senator.

Maureen Buchanan Jones wrote this book and became my friend. Writing this story was a task that could crush even the strong. I know my wife guided me to her. Thank you is not enough. Bob Raser, upon reading this story, became part of the team, and I am extremely grateful for his television and film experience. His video of Maureen's story moved this project to a higher professional level.

Erik and Ryan, my sons, gave me back my life. I would never have made it if not for them. They are each a gift, and there is no day that goes by that I don't feel blessed by their presence.

Maureen Elizabeth Davies Thiel gave me 15 years of love, and she put a promise in my hands. It was an honor to be the soul mate of this selfless woman. I thank her for her life more than anyone will know.

I owe Lisa Neary, now Lisa Thiel, an enormous debt of gratitude for her patience, understanding and love. She is the reason I go on each day.

Finally, I thank all the women that have written to me and said "I thank God for *Maureen's Mission* and what you are doing." That support keeps me focused and reminds me of the need for what I do.

Biographies

William Thiel is a patient advocate for breast cancer. His website, www.maureensmission.org is a referral site for breast cancer questions. His media appearances include the *Martha Stewart Radio Show* and *CNN Headline Newsmakers* and *The State of PA*. Magazines such as *Advanced Radiology and Imaging* have chronicled his work.

Maureen Buchanan Jones, Ph.D., is a free-lance writer and editor of fiction and non-fiction. Her poetry has appeared in *13th Moon,* the *North Dakota Quarterly Review* and *Peregrine.* She leads creative writing workshops and is an Amherst Writers & Artists affiliate. First-hand, personal experiences with cancer are her inherent credentials.

A Promise Fulfilled:

One Couple's Journey Through Misdiagnosis, Breast Cancer and Advocacy

I told my husband, if I live, that's what I'm going to do with my life. I'm going to go around preaching. Doctors can't tell women to go home and don't worry …

Maureen Thiel

I wish I could turn the hands of time back to when I first found this lump.

Maureen Thiel

"What an amazing mission you are fulfilling for your wife. Your love for her is indescribable.… I still have the doctor's message on my answering machine that I did not have cancer. Wow. I did. 5 spots and a mastectomy later, I am doing fabulously … Many thanks for your fine work.

–Nancy G., Letter to Maureen's Mission

I had the surgery and everything was good. I feel great going east to see the grandchildren for the holidays, can't wait. If I hadn't read Maureen's story, I would have never known until it was too late. Thanks for the story."

–Tommie W. Letter to Maureen's Mission

I just wanted to say what a blessing you are for turning such a tragic event in your life into a Gift to all women. I can't thank you enough.

Laurie A. Letter to *Maureen's Mission*

I thank God for Maureen's Mission.
You will never know how many women you will help.

Rebecca T. Letter to *Maureen's Mission*

I want everyone to know I had the pleasure of meeting Maureen Thiel. She was selfless, loving, and caring. This man sitting here in front of you is nothing short of a hero. He is a landscaper, a dad, and A Man on a Mission …

Malcolm MacGregor, Attorney

Introduction

I have learned not to sound angry. I have learned to sound cheerful and positive as I tell an interviewer my reasons for being at a radio or television station. I have learned many things and I use them all to keep the promise I made to my wife to tell her story. I look directly into the camera when they start to film and say: "This story will save your life. You will not hear this story anywhere else, but it is a story that every woman and every woman's daughter needs to hear. When a doctor tells you that you have a breast lump, but 'it's o.k., don't worry,' that's when this story should mean the most to you. It is my wife, Maureen's story, and I promised her that I would tell it as many times as it took to make sure that her story never happens again."

I am a landscaper, a handyman, the guy who shows up with a pick up truck full of lawnmowers and edgers, paint buckets and spackle. I am the guy you call to help pull up some shrubs or remove old wallpaper. I am common sense and can do.

In May of 2006, I sat before CN8 cameras for two pieces that were aired on CNN *Headline Newsmakers*, to educate the viewers on how the lack of standard of care in breast cancer caused my wife's death and thousands of other women as well. I want you to know why it is still happening and what needs to be fixed for patient safety and to maximize the quality of care that is already available to some women, but not all.

As with all disease, breast cancer has a nationally accepted standard of care, which is a set of guidelines for how to identify, diagnose and treat any breast abnormality. It is called "Best Practices for Quality of Care" and was developed by the American Medical Association. Unfortunately, this standard is not enforced by any regulatory agency. Doctors across the country can choose whether to adhere to the national standard or not. Some doctors believe that the correct follow up for a breast lump is to tell their patients: "Don't worry about it. Come back in 6 months or a year." Whereas the nationally accepted standard of care tells doctors that a woman should only wait two menstrual cycles at most, before reassessment. If a lump has not dissipated within that time, a doctor should look at it again. If a woman is post menopausal, 30 days is the maximum wait for a follow up if the lump has not dissipated.

By not following the AMA standards, the doctors who treated her caused my wife, Maureen's death, and this failure is still killing women across this country.

In every interview I give, I repeat that all doctors need to follow the national standard upon which many health care professionals already agree.

I learned this information the hard way. You can learn about the nationally accepted standard of care at www.nccn.org, the National Comprehensive Cancer Network (NCCN) web site along with patient and oncology flow charts. There a woman can educate herself on the right follow up to maximize her safety and forestall a delayed diagnosis.

Every time law suits are brought before a court, the defendants lose when it is proven that they did not follow the national standard of care. In each case the patient who brought the lawsuit is no longer alive or has suffered serious consequences due to the delayed diagnosis of their breast lump. In every case it is proven that a correct follow up according to the national experts could have saved that woman from this silent epidemic. This system is illogical and backward at best, negligent and calloused at worst.

Often, when I am finished talking and the cameras are turned off, the interviewer, the camera crew and the office staff have more questions. Frequently there is someone who has a story similar to Maureen's. I listen and direct them to the sources that will give them the best information available. I have learned how common these stories are. I am still angry, but I have learned not to let it show. Not until I need it, and throughout the last ten years, I have needed my anger. It fuels the work I do. I hone it and direct it until I get the results I want. I never lose my focus.

The names of the doctors in this book have been changed as a way to keep the attention on the important part of the story. This book is not about putting doctors in a bad light or about pointing fingers. This book is about what happens to a woman when she does not have all the facts necessary to be her own best advocate when she finds a lump in her breast. Maureen Thiel did not have all the information she needed to save her life.

This book is our story the way we lived it. I want you to read it so you won't have to. You have the right to an early correct diagnosis. Read this book; educate yourself on the facts, and this will never happen to you or your family. Once the delay has happened, the moment is lost. Maureen could not turn the hands of time back when she first found her lump, but you have her knowledge now. Thank you, from Bill Thiel and Maureen's Mission.

All of my profits will go to Maureen's Mission, a 501C3 non-profit to create public awareness about misdiagnosis and delayed diagnosis, thus saving lives. Profits will also help pay for breast care for the uninsured and underinsured women of this country.

Bill Thiel

Chapter One

Whirlwind

The first time I met Maureen it was two in the morning. It was May and the nights were staying warm the way they do in Florida. I was twenty-three and coming home from a pool tournament. I played pool a lot back then. I had drunk some beer, won't deny that. My good friend Brent and I pulled into his driveway in Tampa, Florida. He lived in a trailer court, the Mighty Grand Trailer Park, or the MGTP, as we called it. I had had enough to drink.

"I'm just going to sleep in my car," I said.

"No, Bill," he said, "I'll see if Shirley will let you sleep on the couch." Shirley is his wife.

So I was sitting there, waiting in the truck, and around the corner came this lady with a dog. I thought to myself, "What's this lady doing walking her dog at 2 a. m.?" I guess my hormones were kicking too, because I got out of the truck. I said something to her like, "Hey, you look good," or "Well, hey, how're you doing'? What's your name?" I don't remember what I said to her really. It wasn't a long conversation. I got back in the truck and waited for Brent to come out. He finally showed, and I said, "Hey, I just met this lady." I described her.

"That's my wife's best friend," he said.

"Man, I'd like to get me some of that."

"Well, you can forget about it, because she's not like that."

I guess it was a challenge or something, I don't know. Next morning, I asked Brent about her again. She was still on my mind.

"You know, last night when I met that lady, I'm not sure if I was rude or anything. Do you know where she lives? I'd like to at least go and apologize." I wasn't a rude person. I never have been. Brent shrugged and told me where she lived and I went and knocked on her door.

"Hi," I said. "I'm Bill. I'm Brent's friend. If I said anything last night that was obnoxious, I'm sorry." I stepped a little closer and caught the smell of her shampoo. I knew I didn't want to let her get away, and all I was thinking was how I wanted to kiss her mouth.

"You didn't say anything to worry about," she said.

She was wearing red shorts and a striped shirt, and I noticed her legs were slim. My head wasn't too clear, so I didn't have anything clever to say. "It was nice meeting you," was all I could think of. So that was the end of that.

At the time, I was doing landscaping work in the mobile home park. Maybe a week later I was doing a mulch job. I worked hard. I also worked in a warehouse driving the flatbeds, so I was pretty strong. I'm not tall or have big muscles, but I'm wiry. I never wore my shirt. I found out later that Maureen was watching me from the window of her trailer. She told her friend Shirley that I had a strong back. "Maureen likes your back," Shirley told me. It made me laugh. But it also made me think I should go over and say 'Hi' to her again. Maybe see if she would go out with me. I always took my yellow lab, Sheba, to the beach, and I knew Maureen had a dog. Maybe she liked the beach. That was my intention when I went over there. I still had the twenty-three-year-old hormone intentions too, don't get me wrong. I'm not going to lie about that.

I did go over to her house, and talked to her and asked her if she liked going to the beach. She went up to the beach all the time too, she said, with Heidi, her Schnauzer. "O.K.," she said. Just like that, 'O.K.'. I picked her up a few days later and we drove about an hour and a half to Sand Key Beach with our dogs. We talked all day long. Just talked about this and that, like two people that don't know each other. I know I did most of the talking. She found out how I'd grown up right around there, even played cork ball right on the lot that was now the trailer park. I told her about the old man who had retired from the circus that used to own the lot. Her eyes just danced when I told her that a tight rope wire and a trampoline used to be where her trailer now stood.

"He had a Coke machine and he'd give all us kids Cokes for free," I said.

"What happened to him? Did he have family?" Maureen asked.

"He died when he was real old. The laundry building in your trailer park was his house."

She laughed and said, "Now I know why I always feel so good when I'm in there folding my towels."

I told her that I moved away from home at 16, and bought my own mobile home at 17 years old. Then I went in the Army for two years. I was on the drop zone ready to go to Iran in the 82nd Air Born in 1979. I got out of the Army in 1981 with an honorable discharge. I told her I lived rent free in a different trailer park while I worked in the warehouse and did landscaping work.

I learned that she had grown up in New Jersey with a younger sister. She told me she and her Dad were close. I watched her as she talked and I couldn't get over the way her smile would come and go. Her face was a slightly long oval with full cheeks and a small chin. Her big, wide smile spread to her cheek bones and then lit up her dark brown eyes like the sun sparkling on deep water. Like the world was a place full of great things. And then Maureen, in her black one-piece bathing suit, stood up with the ocean behind her. I was sitting on the sand looking up at her and something came over me. I don't know what it was, but at that second I knew I was looking at my wife. Don't ask me how I know, I don't know. I just knew it. And it scared me. It really scared me. I'd never felt like that before, so I got quiet. I tried to be polite and make conversation, but now something else was on my mind. I couldn't tell her. I mean, this was the first time we had gone anywhere. During the ride home I kept sneaking glances at her, watching the way her dark hair curled around her face.

When I dropped her off, she said, "Did you have a good time?"

"Yeah, Maureen, I had a great time. It was wonderful."

"Well, you were talking and talking, and then all of a sudden you got quiet. Did I say anything wrong?"

"No, it isn't anything to do with you." But I knew it was. It was everything to do with her. She was going to be my wife and it just scared me.

I couldn't call her after that. I told my friends, but I don't think they understood. I think you can only understand if something like that has happened to you. And I've heard of it happening to people like that, where you just know. In the movie, *Sleepless in Seattle,* Tom Hanks does a great job explaining how it just happens. It's magic. But I was too afraid to call her back. I wanted to see her again. Of course I wanted to see her again. I just didn't know how or when.

A few weeks later I was doing another job in the trailer court and Maureen saw me; my truck was there, and she purposely went around the long way. I know, because I wasn't working on the way to the exit. She pulled up in her car, rolled her window down and said, "Hi, how've you been?"

"Hi. O.K., I guess." My mouth went kind of dry.

"Oh," she said, "I just thought you didn't like me, you know. You said you had a good time, but I haven't heard from you."

I leaned on my shovel and swallowed. "I was going to call you, Maureen, you know, I just, you know, I was going to call you …" I knew she was a beautician from all our conversation at the beach. "Do you cut hair on the side?"

"Yeah, I cut hair," she said, kind of like a question.

"Well I need a hair cut. Could you cut my hair?"

"All right, come on over Friday evening when you're done working. I'll be done working too, and I'll cut your hair then."

On the way to her house I stopped and got a bottle of wine. It's not everyday you get a bottle of wine to go get a hair cut. This was going to be the day that I told her what I felt at the beach. I had to tell her. When I got there, we had a couple of glasses of wine and she started to cut my hair. We talked a little about the trailer park, Shirley and Brent, the dogs. Then she asked me if I was good at school.

"I did o.k., but mostly because I never had to write down things like vocabulary words. I've always been good at remembering details. I read people well too. That's always helped me." Then I got quiet again, thinking about how I was reading her.

Maureen put down the scissors. "You're quiet again Bill, just like you were at the beach."

All I saw were her eyes, big and brown, full of questions. "Is there something wrong?" she asked.

I looked in her eyes and I said, "Maureen, I've got something to tell you." I don't know what she thought, but I said, "You're going to be my wife." How many people do you meet one time and then they come to your house the next time and tell you, "You're going to be my wife." She looked at me without saying a word. All I saw were her eyes, and her eyes said, "I know."

I stood up and put my arms around her. I could feel our hearts touching beneath the skin. We were both quiet and I didn't know what else to say, so I said good-bye and I gave her another hug. She just took it all in.

I walked out to my truck. I got in my truck. I put my key in the ignition and started the truck. I shut it off. I got out. I went back to the door and knocked. I said, "Maureen, I have to spend some time with you."

She nodded and held the door open for me. I wanted her in my arms so badly. I knew she wanted that too. I knew that. But I had to tell her. "Maureen," I said. "I'm never going to have sex with you."

She didn't say anything.

"Maureen, I'm always going to make love to you." When we went to bed that night I just held her. If you could feel two bodies become one, that's what happened. I never left her from that day.

The very next day I gathered up my stuff and moved right in with her. We fit together no matter what we did. One of the things we always liked was to go to amusement parks. Sometimes we wouldn't even ride; we'd walk around watching people, laughing at our own jokes and feeling the air that we shared moving around us. If we did go on rides, there was one Maureen would never get on. She was afraid of roller coasters. I'd go on and she'd stand and watch, grinning at me as I spun by. She wasn't afraid of much, but she wouldn't touch roller coasters.

Maureen was a gift. The best gift that anyone ever got times 20 million isn't as good as the gift I got. She was born Maureen Elizabeth Davies on February 3, 1955 in Elizabeth, New Jersey, the older of two girls. Davies is a Welsh name and you pronounce it 'Davis.' Her parents were George and Margaret, and her sister was Katheryn. She grew up in a one-story brick house with window boxes and a little framed in pool in the back yard. On her second birthday she got a crown and a peddle car. Later her family made trips to Ozone Park and the beach; they went camping and on vacations to places like Cape Cod and Ontario. She grew to be 5'3" tall and never weighed more than 130 pounds. In high school she fell in love with the Beatles, took the usual algebra and English classes as well as a half-day set of courses at a vocational school to learn to be a beautician.

It was in sewing class in tenth grade at Cranford High that Maureen met her best friend Lynn Salerno. Unlike Maureen, Lynn wasn't much for craft-type things and she got her finger stuck under the needle trying to push a piece of cloth through. Maureen thought it was hilarious and raised the needle so Lynn could pull her finger out. They were true friends from then on. They were home base for each other. "With Maureen I don't have to cover the time when we don't see each other. We just pick up where we left off," Lynn always said. Lynn even went into hairdressing just because of Maureen, but it was Maureen that really took to it and had the talent.

Maureen graduated in 1973 with a high school diploma and a certificate as a hairdresser. It was exactly what she wanted to be. She worked in high school, cutting hair and doing perms. When she graduated, she kept on working in New Jersey for a few years, and never had trouble finding good jobs.

She and Lynn went to clubs, danced all night, flirted with boys. They rode around listening to Bruce Springsteen, Steely Dan, and The Cars. Lynn used to say to me, "Maureen always finds excitement, because she sees it everywhere around her. She makes her own fun." But it was also because Maureen never put conditions on their friendship and took most everybody on their own terms. The only person from high school that Lynn stayed in touch with was Maureen. Sometimes they'd argue, but they always worked it out, and Maureen would say to Lynn, "Who loves ya, baby?"

When Lynn turned eighteen, Maureen, a year older, threw her a surprise party. When Lynn opened the door, everyone yelled, "Surprise!" Lynn was surprised all right. She didn't recognize anyone. They were all guys. Maureen just stood there laughing. "Lynn," she said, "I figured we'd definitely get lucky tonight. We have no competition!" The two girls went to the Bahamas soon after and had a blast. Lynn and Maureen were inseparable.

Right around that time, Maureen found a lump in her left breast. Her mom took her right away to the doctor and had it removed. It turned out to be a cyst and Maureen never worried about it again. She did her breast exams the way she was taught in health class.

After a few years of working in New Jersey, Maureen got a chance to work as a hairdresser on a cruise ship out of Cape Canaveral, Florida in 1981. She always wanted to see what the world offered and never settled for ordinary. She worked for six months then met an Englishman on one of the cruises. He must have swept her away, because they were married within two weeks. They went to London to meet his family, and then Maureen and that first Bill got an apartment in New Jersey. Lynn suspected that he was rough with Maureen, and soon, he insisted that they move to Florida. He told Maureen to borrow money, so Maureen went to Lynn.

Maureen never borrowed or lent money, so Lynn was suspicious.

"Bill wants to move." Maureen told her. "It's for him I'm asking."

"I can't give it you," Lynn said. "If it was for you, I'd give you anything you needed. You know that."

Maureen and Bill moved to Florida anyway, and right after that he left her. Maureen knew then he'd married her to get a green card. When she called Lynn, all she said was, "I have to figure this out." No whining or feeling sorry. Maureen always took responsibility for her own decisions, even if they didn't work out. They got divorced no more than six months after they had gotten married. That's all she ever told me.

I met Maureen in May of 1983, and we got married in Christ Chapel at the corner of Skipper Road and Livingston Avenue right across from the MGTP on March 31, 1984. The Chapel was one of those old, white clapboard churches you see on calendars of New England. It was set on five acres with a little parsonage house next to it. It didn't seat more than fifty people, but it held all our happiness. It wasn't a big wedding, but that didn't mean Maureen didn't give it all her attention. She planned every bit of it herself. She wore a straight white satin dress with lace at the top. Instead of a veil, she wore a white hat with a wide brim that made her look happy and sexy at the same time. I'll never forget seeing her eyes, dark and shining as she looked at me and said, "I do." I was half a person when I met my wife and she was half a person. Together we were one. We went on a cruise to Nassau on our honeymoon and when we got back we stood on the deck of the ship in Port Canaveral and saw the shuttle take off. I know, "rockets going off".

We bought an acre of property, 2805 Olavet Court, in Valrico, Florida, with one tree and a dumpy mobile home. The trailer was so bad the kitchen sink fell through the counter top the second week after we moved in. I got busy evenings after work, and between the two of us, we fixed that place up so it was just great. Maureen painted the new kitchen cabinets a dark teal with white trim. Country ducks lined the window sill and a sign that said, "God bless our home," hung near the fridge. She was in her glory decorating, picking out curtains, and putting up pictures. She liked gardening too. She was a homebody and never asked for more than a clean place to make her own and share with the people she loved.

I got my landscaping business going and pretty soon we had over a hundred trees and just as many shrubs planted everywhere in our yard. I planted Leyland cypress trees, holly bushes, sweet gum maples and crepe myrtles. After a while the business included two landscape trucks with four employees in the winter and seven in the summer. I worked 80 hours a week. Maureen worked cutting hair at Rita's Salon in Valrico.

Lynn came down to visit and she couldn't believe it. "When you told me you lived in a mobile home, I pictured something a lot different than this," she confessed. Maureen laughed and showed her the flowers she had planted and how she had painted, stenciled and put up wallpaper. I think it puzzled Lynn to see Maureen so content. But Maureen wasn't so much a contradiction as a well-rounded person. She made her own party wherever she was, even when it was making a home out of a mobile trailer.

After we got married I still couldn't wait to get home to Maureen after work. One of the first evenings, she turned to me in the kitchen and gave me a sweet hug. I knew right then that's what I wanted every day after work. "Let me help you get dinner ready," I said, not wanting to be away from her.

"Don't you want to go in and watch T.V.? Relax or something? You just got home from work," she asked me.

"I might be done for the day, but you're still working." I took the chopping knife out of her hand and started in on the carrots. She stood for a minute, her head to one side watching me. She gave a little sigh, like settling into something that made her feel good, and she got the lettuce from the fridge and washed it in the sink.

We sat at the table and I told her about the guys teasing me that I was too married and should go with them for beers after work.

"You should go," she said. "I don't want you to lose your friends."

I took her hands, soft, with pretty nails. Mine felt like sandpaper claws from handling dirt and stone all day. "I'm not going to lose any friends. But I sure as hell am not going to lose you over some guys." She laughed, but I meant it.

"I'm not going anywhere," she said. "I'll be right here when you get home." She stood up to clear the plates.

I followed her to the sink with the rest of the dishes. "Hey, maybe if I wash these my hands will soften up. That'll be my nighttime beauty routine." She laughed pretty hard at that one, but she didn't' stop me from filling the sink with suds and scrubbing the dishes. She dried and we talked more about what we wanted to do to the house. We kept that routine every night of our marriage.

When I first met Maureen, I played on a championship softball team. We practiced on Sunday mornings and the rule was, if you don't practice, you don't play. After a few months of my getting up and going off every Sunday morning, Maureen told me flat out she didn't like it.

"Sunday morning is the only morning of the week I get to spend with you," she said. "Every other morning we both have to get up and get going to work. I miss you on Sunday."

I could have argued with her. I had a lot of fun playing on that team, and I liked winning. But I liked spending time with her too. Maureen loved to have me hold her. When I married her I told her she was more important than anything else. So I quit, and I spent Sunday mornings loving Maureen. You could call it a disagreement, but I never really thought twice about changing my life for her.

Don't get me wrong, we had our disagreements. It's just that they were so small we forgot about them the next day. One thing that drove me crazy was how Maureen was always late. It wasn't because she lost track of time or didn't care, but because she had to make sure everything was perfect before she left the house. She checked her hair, her lipstick, the windows, the knobs on the stove and the locks on the doors. Sometimes she had to do it twice. I'd sit in the car steaming, and then she'd come out with her big smile. Mostly I let it go. We both let the small stuff go and had fun being together. Maybe it was because we both knew we wanted something different from the way we had grown up.

I grew up in a trailer, one of six kids. Some nights we all huddled in a pit we had dug under the trailer and listened to my dad beat on my mom. They both drank. Maureen grew up on a suburban street with small brick houses, but things weren't always happy there either. Her mom was depressed a lot, and Maureen didn't always hear the love that a kid needs to hear. We both missed something when we were kids, and we found it in each other.

We lived in Florida from 1984 to 1991. Maureen always took good care of herself. She had learned from her junior high health teacher how to check her body for any changes. She did a breast exam every month in the shower and she got full check ups every year just like she was supposed to.

We didn't know it, but the best times were still to come when the boys were born. Maureen couldn't have loved those two kids more. She lived for them. But the first time she got pregnant, she miscarried while she was at work. The doctor told her to go home and rest for a while. She went back to work after a few days and within a few months she was pregnant again. The doctor told her if she could afford to stay off her feet, she should. Maureen knew I was working as hard as I could and that we needed the extra money, but I told her not to worry. Her job was to start being a mom right then. I went to all her appointments with her, so I would know right away what we needed to do to keep Maureen healthy and take care of the baby.

Everything went great with Maureen's pregnancy. She ate like pregnant ladies do, but she walked and followed orders.

"It's time to walk the Mom," I'd say to her.

"Yeah, well, right now, I feel like the Mom could use a wheelbarrow."

I started laughing.

"What? What's so funny?"

"Maureen, you've got two different shoes on!"

"Well, I can't reach my feet." Now she really started laughing. "And I can't see them either."

The baby must have known he had a good spot, because the due date came and went without a peep. Then a week went by and still nothing happened. Finally, it was sixteen days past the due date and Maureen was looking like the baby and the June heat were going to flatten her even when she wasn't moving. Maureen's dad and sister came to help out. They were just pulling into the driveway at about 6:30 in the evening, when a small tornado touched down at the far edge of our property. I gave a whoop and got them into the garage. I heard a whoop from Maureen inside, because all her knick-knacks were rattling off the shelves. It was only a few hours later at about 10:30 when she went into labor. We always laughed and said it took a tornado to get that baby born.

We got to the hospital and Maureen started in on breathing right and pushing, but she wasn't dilating no matter what. I gave her ice and back rubs and walked her up and down the hall. The doctors put on music, so Maureen could try a little slow dancing to get things moving. Nothing. At this point, the monitor showed the baby was in distress, so the doctor set her up for a C-section. I stood on the surgeon's side and watched everything, the little head and shoulders rising out of Maureen's belly while the Moody Blues played in the background.

Maureen's medical records at this point were routine, but I'm including them from this point on because they are a critical part of this story. They are taken verbatim from her doctors' reports and will appear as inserts. At first the medical records show only small concerns, and they appear within the story just the way a doctor's visit happens within the normal course of every day activities. As the story unfolds, the medical records will describe in the doctors' own words how Maureen's health changed and how each doctor responded.

Summary: Routine doctors visits and birth of Erik
Medical Records 1986-1991
Had routine pelvic examinations with Pap smears each year.
6/23/86 delivered Erik by C-section. Breast fed.

Erik was born on June 23, 1986. Maureen had a scar from the Caesarean section, but nothing made her happier than holding that baby. I had my own landscaping company by this time and was real busy, so Maureen took to being a mom; she was so proud of her baby. She nursed him and followed all of the pediatrician's advice.

For Erik's first birthday there must have been twenty kids and twice as many adults. In the video of that day, Maureen is wearing a red sundress with blue and yellow triangles. She moves in her easy way, hugging a neighbor wife or helping a kid carry their present into the house. She gathers the kids around the table. Every one of them has on a pointy party hat and they all sing. Maureen bends over Erik and helps him blow out the candle. She cuts the cake and serves ice cream, letting Erik go at his piece with his hands until he's a sticky mess. The room is full of people, light and air.

Almost two years later, on March 30, 1988, Maureen gave me another son and Erik a little brother, Ryan. For Ryan, the doctors just scheduled a C-section, because they didn't want to take any chances. It was kind of weird to have an appointment at 9 or 10 o'clock to go have a baby. But have a baby we did. While Maureen was in the hospital she made friends with Cheryl Allsup. Cheryl's daughter was born the same day as Ryan, and Maureen and Cheryl hung out all the time after that. Cheryl was a nurse, so she was very helpful with breast feeding or if the kids ran a fever or got a cold.

Summary: Birth of Ryan
Medical Record 3/30/88
Delivered Ryan by C-section & a tubal ligation at same time.
Breast fed.

Maureen picked out both names for the boys; I listened to her ideas and let her tell me the names of my sons. Watching her, I felt like she was doing what she had been waiting to do all her life. Maureen had her tubes tied during that C-section. We had our two boys and Maureen had the family she always wanted. I still couldn't believe this woman was there waiting for me every night.

By 1990 we had the house and yard in Valrico looking pretty good and the boys were two and four. Maureen would fill up the plastic pool for dark-haired Erik and blond Ryan and let them splash and jump. I can still see her lying on the chaise lounge in her two-piece black and white bathing suit. She is tanning her back with her straps undone and Ryan dumps a bucket of water on her shoulders.

She holds her top and rolls up onto her side, her big smile beaming on Ryan. "No more water on Mommy, Ryan. Pour the water in the pool."

He goes back to the pool, scoops another bucket and runs back to dump it on her again. They are both laughing. Erik is jumping up and down in the pool. Maureen ties her bathing suit top and stands, her hands on her hips and shakes her thick curls at the boys. Ryan pours the water on her feet, Erik shrieks and they both jump in and out of the pool. Maureen watches, her eyes filled with everything she wants. When she realizes I'm there with the camera pointed at her, she rolls her eyes. When I do a close up of her breasts, she gives a self-deprecating laugh in her throat and turns away, but I know she is pleased by the way she tosses her hair.

Later we watch the boys on the slip and slide.

"Look at Ryan, he never stops moving and Erik never gives up."

We have made a family, a family like the one we each wanted when we were kids. She never veered from that job.

A lot of weekends we went to Sand Key Beach. She wore plaid shorts and a white sleeveless top as she unpacked peanut butter and jelly sandwiches and poured Kool-Aid from the orange thermos jug into paper cups. The boys wore dark swim trunks with yellow water wings around each of their puny biceps. Maureen made sure the valves were shut tight and wouldn't lose air. Then she pulled off her shorts and shirt and waded into the big rolling waves, letting them hit her thighs as the wind caught her hair. The curves of her body matched the curves of the rising and falling ocean. She turned and watched the boys for a moment, then moved steadily into the surf until she was thigh deep. She looked like she was taking in the whole ocean through her pores; her gaze wide and focused far out on the horizon. She rose slightly as the waves swelled up and over her belly. She looked back once and waved, then turned, waited for a wave to rise behind her then dove and let the wave carry her until it broke. Erik threw down his shovel and ran into the surf toward her.

We attended the First Presbyterian Church every Sunday. The boys wore creased trousers and white and black shoes shined each Saturday afternoon. Maureen had a Sunday dress that was my favorite, I called it her gypsy dress. It was white with a flounce at the top that she wore just slightly down on her shoulders. The skirt flared into a big circle that swayed when she moved. In her ears were white hoop earrings. The first time I saw it, I said, "You look too good to be going to church."

She came close and kissed me. "I wouldn't dress any different for God than I do for you."

I watched her walk up the aisle and sit in the pew, her head up, her back straight, her eyes and mind on the Lord, holding Ryan by the hand. She wasn't playing games with God; she was talking right to him with her heart. I know God was listening. He even sent us a whirlwind.

One afternoon when Erik was about four and Ryan must have been two, we were all out in the yard, the boys climbing around on the ladder for the swing set, Maureen planting salvia and I was washing down one of the trucks. It was a sunny day, calm, probably about 92 degrees, when all of a sudden I saw this whirlwind set down over in the corner by the cypress trees. Maureen saw it too, but neither of us said a word. Maureen picked up Ryan and I grabbed Erik by the hand, and we ran towards it. We stepped inside, wide eyed. It was about five feet across at the base and moved across the yard at a walking pace. We followed where it was going by watching the grass whip in circles.

Maureen's sundress kept blowing up around her waist. She pulled it down with one hand while she had Ryan on her hip. We were both laughing real hard. I put my arm in the edge of it and felt the wind sucking past and leaves rattling against my skin. Maureen did it too and then Erik did. Maureen took Ryan's arm and put it in the wind. He clung to Maureen, tilted his face up to her and grinned at her with his eyes wide. The whirlwind picked up speed, and we had to do a kind of two-step to keep up with it. We followed it for a 100 or 125 feet before it suddenly went straight up into the sky. Erik jumped up to catch it, and Ryan waved good-by. Maureen and I stood there grinning. There's not an amusement ride in the world that has ever compared with that whirlwind.

But our ordinary days were pretty good too. Our house was the meeting place for all our friends and neighbors. We had barbecues and parties. I built a bonfire pit out of railroad ties. After the holidays the neighbors brought their Christmas trees over. We put on music, put the beer on ice, started up the grills and watched the trees burn.

Routine doctors visits
Medical Record 1990
Was treated and biopsied for Dysfunctional Uterine Bleeding.
Endometrial and endocervical biopsies were negative.
No breast complaints noted throughout these records.

Medical Record 5/31/91
Baseline Mammogram
"Moderate fibrous stromal tissue without evidence of dominant mass lesion or pathologic calcifications."

On weekends we played. Just because we had the boys didn't mean we stopped going to amusement parks. We just went to a different kind. Maureen and I took Erik and Ryan to Al's Wonderland near Valrico. It was a small, family-owned place with train rides, bumper boats and go-carts for little kids. They loved it! But I think Maureen loved it even more. She took them to each ride and coaxed them behind the steering wheel and strapped them in, then stood back and watched what they'd do. She stood by the railing just eating them up with her eyes, taking in their determined faces, the way they grabbed the steering wheels, the way Ryan enjoyed just being in a boat and Erik liked being in control. She never directed them to be different than they were.

When the boys were old enough, she put them into a little pre-school that was part of our church, and she joined the Westminster Academy Day Care mother's group to do fund-raising and help organize activities for the kids. The mother's group had guest speakers who gave talks on subjects, like how to get your kids to sleep through the night, or how to manage working and parenting. Maureen came home after one meeting and said a woman in her 30's had spoken about breast cancer. This woman had just had a mastectomy, and it shocked Maureen. "She was so young, Bill. She told us it could happen to anyone." It scared her and reinforced her commitment to get yearly breast exams.

By 1991, my landscaping business was doing well. I had plenty of work and people in the area knew I could be trusted. But Maureen's Dad, George was having a hard time making the trip from New Jersey down to Valrico for visits. He had open-heart surgery and then developed lung cancer. Maureen wanted to be closer so the boys could spend time with their grandfather. I closed up the business, we packed up everything and moved to northeast Pennsylvania.

We found a house to rent in the Pocono Mountain Lake Estates in Bushkill, and right away we felt at home. The development sits right next to the Delaware Water Gap Recreation Area. Only a few miles to the north is the Delaware National Forest. Old stone walls run through old fields that are now succeeding into young white pines, white oaks and maples. The land rises and dips, with small lanes that curve and angle to give views into a continuous series of small valleys with fast running streams. In the spring, freshets bubble up throughout the landscape and deer run across the yards every day. I saw a mountain lion once just at dusk.

The development was put up in the 1980s and most of the houses are two to four bedrooms with just one or one and a half baths. The house we rented was small, but typical, just a modular ranch. Most of the homes were probably about 1,400 square feet. Some were bigger where families had added on. There were a few larger homes and these were the newer ones, the ones where people bought lots and built on them. The development was a mix of families who lived there year round and folks from New York City or New Jersey who were here for weekend or summer getaways.

The dues per year were $500. That fee included the expectation that we would do volunteer work. I helped build the lakefront beach pavilion and the volleyball sand pit. The community also had a million dollar community center with an outdoor pool, tennis courts, horseshoe pit, barbecue and picnic grounds, and baseball diamonds. The clubhouse held an indoor pool and sauna, fireplace, pool tables, recreation room for the kids, and a large function room with a bar and dance floor.

It sounds exclusive, but it was home to regular people. We thought it would be great for the boys and for us. The neighborhood association spent thousands of dollars on the kids. We made great friends because it was a community of wonderful people. Maureen used to say it was like living on a cruise ship. Every week we'd get a sheet of activities for the kids, and all summer long there were picnics, barbeques, and even a little Olympics.

The kids went sledding in our back yard in the winter; we were right in the foothills of the Pocono Mountains. The boys tumbled and rolled right down the hill in the back and learned to swerve around the trees. In the winter, with all the leaves down, we could see Kittatinny Mountain and further to the south, Jenny Jump Mountain in New Jersey. In the summer we could hear a waterfall not far from the house.

Neither one of us had a job when we got to Bushkill, so I took a paper route, and Maureen got a part-time job in a grocery store. Within a few months I found a job with a pharmaceutical company working the night shift pulling orders. I worked at that for a few more months until I answered an ad for a job with Steve Willand, Distributor of Power and Outdoor Equipment. Even through the part-time jobs, I always made sure we had health insurance. Maureen's miscarriage made me careful about that.

Every day, my route to work took me over Dingmans Bridge, the oldest privately owned bridge in the United States. It's part of Rte. 209 and is the only way across the Delaware River unless you drive all the way up to Milford or even further down to East Stroudsburg. It's a wooden trestle bridge that costs 75¢ each way. One of the owners stands at the tollbooth on the Pennsylvania side and collects the money. It's barely wide enough for two cars, and the wooden roadway thumps and clacks as you roll across. Right here the Delaware is usually calm and slow with rugged banks sloping up on either side. The bridge sits in the middle of the Delaware National Park. Once across the bridge, you are in the town of Lawton, New Jersey. Bushkill felt like coming home for us and most of that feeling came from the neighbors.

The first time Maureen met her friends Patty Flotz, Helen Sheffo and Laurie Zuchino was up at the lake during a barbecue. All the families gathered at the pool during the day or up at the lake in the evenings. Maureen was usually right in the middle of the woman, talking and laughing. Maureen and Patty just hit it off right way. They had kids and family in common, and Patty told me Maureen was easy to get to know. Maureen cut all the Flotz's hair.

Maureen loved going to the lake in her jeans and sweatshirt to watch the boys swim. She always had something to keep her hands busy, or they'd be moving in front of her as she talked. They'd get going real fast when she was excited. Maureen fit right into the Pocono Mountain community. She made ashtrays for the lake. She painted coffee cans, decorated them and filled them with sand to help keep the place clean. She also started the Christmas cookie exchange. It was just another way to share. But mostly it was about the kids and ordinary concerns. Once in a while a crisis pulled everybody together.

When Erik was six, he got burned on the 4th of July weekend, 1992. I had climbed on top of the lake pavilion to hang a flag, and I heard him yell. He was down below looking at his foot one second, and then he took off to the water the next. Someone had dropped hot coals into the sand near the pavilion and covered them over with sand. I jumped off the pavilion, and Maureen, who was at the end of the beach with Ryan, started running. We met in the water. Erik's foot and leg had just melted. Maureen went wild. Everybody wanted us to wait for an ambulance, but Maureen said, "No way. We're taking him now."

The traffic on Route 209 was tied up all along the road for eight miles. It's one lane each way, so even on regular weekdays it's congested. Maureen sat in the back with Erik. She put ice into a cooler and put his leg in it, and I drove with my flashers on, blowing the horn. When we got to the hospital, we found out he had third degree burns.

I took time off from work to help take care of Erik who needed saline baths several times a day. It was hard for Maureen to care of the two boys, and it really upset her to see his leg like that. Neighbors and friends told us to sue the community for negligence, so we filed papers and received a check for $150 to compensate for bandages and saline solution. Maureen called her dad. He told her to mail the check right back, not to cash it, not to do anything.

Patty and Rob Flotz had a big barbecue a few weeks later. Rob had a ponytail back then and everyone took bets to get him to cut it off. They made $100 and gave it to us to help pay for Erik's bandages. You can't get better friends than that. Erik had to have several surgeries over the next two years for skin grafts. When the settlement finally came, Erik got financial compensation that he would receive in stages. Maureen and I got $14,000 as compensation for bandages and for loss of wages.

That November Rob Flotz and I, along with a couple of other guys, sold Christmas trees for extra money. Maureen, Helen, Laurie and Patty made wreaths from the trimmed branches. Everyone worked during the day, so we set up the stand at night and on weekends. We got trees from a supplier west of Bushkill and sold them on Petrizzo's lot on Rte. 209. Maureen made ornaments and decorations and sold them along with the Christmas trees. We had so much fun, talking to the people that came by, helping them pick out the right tree and drinking the hot chocolate or coffee that Maureen and her friends made. Maureen's joy could have lit up those trees without ever stringing lights on them.

The following Christmas Maureen and I made wooden reindeers with little lights around the antlers. I built them and Maureen sanded and painted them. We named them and gave one to each of our friends. The Flotzes got Blitzen. They still put him out on the lawn and light him up every Christmas.

When we first got to Bushkill, we attended the Presbyterian Church. About 1996, we visited the Reformed Church of Bushkill, an interdenominational community-based church. About fifteen families prayed together with a minister named Isaac, and then stayed for breakfast. Afterwards, the kids played ball in the yard while all the grown-ups talked. It suited us just right. We believed standard, main line Protestant doctrine. Not so different from other churches.

We worked hard to bring in new members and soon we had over a hundred families in our congregation. It still wasn't a large church, but there was a special spirit that brought everybody together. We were proud of our church and that transition. We were there for one another and willing to work to keep the church going. You could feel it every Sunday.

The church itself was built in 1832, but it had burned and was rebuilt in 1872. It's a plain, white clapboard church with a high steeple and thin, arched stained glass windows all in the same pattern. The stained glass is pale rose and blue with a simple Victorian design. Underneath one back window, a plaque reads 'In memory of our daughter, Mary G. Kooms. 1899–1918. Maureen pointed that out to me the first day we went. "It's like we're still praying for her," she said. "That feels like family." Curved, dark oak pews gave us a simple, gracious place to worship. The church steeple has a bell we rang every Sunday. Downstairs, in the community room, round tables sat six.

People packed into the little fellowship hall after service with lots of food and everybody catching up with each other. Sometimes it was hard getting people out of here. We met great people, like Steve and Jennifer Schoonover and their son Jonathan. They were both retired schoolteachers who owned Outdoor Power Equipment and sold generators all over the county. Jennifer has the prettiest smile and gives the best hugs. Steve too, every time you see him. Even at fifty or so, they were still in love. Jennifer used to say, "We're partners all the way." Jonathan was my cooking buddy at the church. I used to put eggs in Jonathan's pocket and then smash them. It would make us laugh so hard, we'd nearly burn everything else cooking on the stove.

I saw Marina Cameron, the Church Administrator, watching us one Sunday. I went over and said, "What are you looking at, Marina?" I was teasing her. But she said, "Maureen is always smiling, and your family looks so happy. If you had had a 75-year marriage, I don't think it would be long enough. I can see the love, respect, and tenderness."

We went about our lives, working and raising our two boys. I kept finding different jobs, each time a little more money, a little better health insurance. Maureen worked at the grocery store and put in a few days at a beauty parlor. A lot of days, I'd just be getting in from work and Maureen would be heading out to the shop. We were like most families I know, juggling our time to pay the mortgage and spend time with the kids.

Maureen used to do an imitation of me on the phone. "This is Bill," she'd say. "Yeah, I can do that," make a note, "I can do that, I can do that."

I'd start at 5 a.m. and go until 10 p.m. She'd ask me "How can you do all that?" Then she'd tell friends when they would ask if I could do a small handyman job, "Bill can do all that. I don't know how he can, but he can."

The boys did fine in school. Erik was the quiet one and kept a bit to himself. Ryan was always talking. They both loved their Mom's company. Maureen was at the center of everything. If I came home and didn't find anyone there, I knew where to look. There was always something going on up at the clubhouse, so Maureen took the boys up there lots of afternoons. Friday or Saturday nights we'd meet friends there and play pool while the kids played ping pong or hung out with friends. They'd beg for money for sodas and ask to have a sleep over. Maureen almost always said yes.

I was the bartender at many of the clubhouse functions with Maureen's help. If there was dancing, she was right there. She could cut a rug all night long. She'd have a beer or a glass of wine; at Christmas it would be peach schnapps, and she'd dance to Frank Sinatra songs or boogey to the Temptations. But when a song came on that she could twist to, that always got her up on the floor. At home it was country music. LeAnn Rimes was her favorite.

Maureen was a big camper too. She took the boys to Promise Land State Park for two weeks in the summer when I had to work. I came on the weekends. If it wasn't Promise Land it might be Knoebles Amusement Park or Dorny Park. In the winter it might be a trip up the road to Fernwood, a timeshare resort, where Maureen and the boys went sledding. Once we went to Gettysburg to learn about the Civil War. Often, even when I was busy with work, Maureen took the boys by herself.

I think she was happiest when she was surrounded by nothing but trees and the smell of clean air. When we got to the campsite, Maureen had a routine, just like she did at home. First she cleaned the spot where the tent would go. She raked out all the rocks and twigs to smooth the ground. She even made little pathways. Setting up the tent was the next thing. It was a six-person tent, with two separate rooms and a little front room. It took some maneuvering to set up, but Maureen was good at it and she made it fun for the kids. We didn't use air mattresses, just sleeping bags with a few blankets underneath.

Maureen brought hot dogs, cheeseburgers, peanut butter, chips and *YooHoo* for the boys. I think they're still stuck on *YooHoo* from their camping days. Sometimes she brought plastic bottles of *Kool-Aid*. We had campfires, of course, and we toasted marshmallows. Once in a while we did s'mores.

During the day we went swimming in the lake or fishing from a rented boat. Maureen liked swimming, but she wasn't much for fishing so she sat in the sun, reading magazines, a Nora Roberts novel or one of those *Chicken Soup* books. One time she surprised Erik and Ryan with two nice bikes. She and I had old bikes that she brought along too. We went for ten-mile bike rides around the lake with a packed picnic lunch or a stop at an ice cream place right along the road. We did that every time, and the boys loved it.

Maureen's favorite thing in late July and August at Promise Land was to go blueberry and raspberry picking. The wild raspberries were the sweetest. We picked for hours and she always yelled at me for eating too many. "Bill, there's not going to be enough for pies," she'd say. Then she'd laugh and throw one at me to see if I could catch it in my mouth. I'd make blueberry pancakes the next morning over the campfire while Maureen slept in a bit. She said those were the best breakfasts she ever had.

In 1994, after renting for those first years, we saved up enough to buy a house right in the Pocono Mountain Lake Estates. It wasn't big or fancy, just a house where you could raise two boys, have friends in to relax, and talk over problems at the kitchen table. It was only a two-bedroom house, so Erik and Ryan shared a room. There were Ninja turtle sheets for Ryan, and Ghost Buster sheets for Erik. Maureen put up a shelf for Ryan's monkey collection. Every special occasion she gave him a stuffed monkey until there were 74 all around the room. I even fixed up a little room in the basement for her like a salon.

She cut our friends' hair and did perms and charged two dollars for a cut. She felt bad the day she had to raise her price to three dollars because the cost of her shampoos and perm solutions went up. Everybody came to her, and not just because she did a good job for cheap. Whenever she had somebody down there, I heard all kinds of laughing going on. If it was quiet, I knew somebody was telling Maureen something hard. Maureen cut hair at other people's houses too, people that couldn't get down their stairs, older people. She brought, and probably spent more on the food than she made for the hair cut.

The money Maureen earned was food money. She clipped coupons and matched up what we needed with what was on sale every week. Once in a while she bought a piece of pottery from the Bushkill Market: heavy bowls and covered jars with blue speckle rims and a blade of wheat on each one. That pottery was like her art collection. She said it made her feel peaceful to see it sitting on her hutch.

She went every week to Albee's grocery store, because it had good discounts and the boys went with her. If she was in a good mood, she let them run around the aisles and build pyramids out of cans, but never so they bothered anyone. Maureen was stern about how the boys behaved in public.

When the boys were nine and eleven, they were supposed to help her carry the groceries in from the car. They were fooling around and Erik lost his hold on the bag. It slipped, smashing the milk on the walkway. There was no going back to the store for more milk. It was too far, and the money was spent. Maureen sent both of the boys to their room.

Often, I'd come home and find out that one or both of them had gotten into trouble. At first they tried to hide it from Maureen. But she would find out and make them sit in their rooms. To a kid it probably seemed like an eternity. I snuck in Oreos and listened to what happened; their mom never let them have chocolate before dinner. They complained about being punished, but they knew their mom was right. Maureen was the law in our house.

Homework was always done as soon as the kids came home from school. Maureen was tough on that, because it was important to her that they get a good education. The boys came home and found her in jeans, a flowered sweatshirt with the sleeves rolled up and Garth Brooks or Shania Twaine on the radio, pushing the vacuum around and singing "*Whose bed have your boots been under*"? at the top of her lungs.

Or she folded the wash and asked questions about what happened at school. If it was a rainy day and none of the boys' friends were coming over, Maureen played board games with them before dinner. The boys didn't do chores except keep their rooms clean. Maureen cleaned the rest of the house.

Both boys, but especially Ryan liked going downstairs and watching Maureen cut hair. She didn't mind. She let them sit on a stool and listen in to the news from around the neighborhood or the church. She cut the kids hair too. When Ryan was six he asked for a Mohawk, so she did it. He was so proud of that. And Maureen was proud of her boys. She ran the house like clockwork and managed to keep everyone healthy. She never missed a yearly checkup.

Routine doctor visit
Medical Record 4/25/94
No breast complaints.
Breast exam listed as within normal limits. Intake sheet reads "cysts on breasts years ago." Mammogram is suggested as the record reads "never had a mammogram."

We didn't have a lot, our home was small, but Maureen went to craft shows and got ideas for decorating the house. If she had an idea, she got the drill, the level, the molly screws and went to work. Maureen could grab a paintbrush or put on the work gloves and work right beside me. She helped move boulders. Maureen made the house comfortable so visitors felt like taking their shoes off and staying for a visit.

She went to yard sales and had a way of picking things out for cheap and making them look good, even her clothes. Maureen didn't care about designer clothes or fancy labels. She shopped at K-mart and Wal-Mart because she thought the money was better spent on Erik or Ryan or on something for the family. But everything she wore was crispy clean and pressed. Her white shirts were white, white. She even ironed her blue jeans. Her clothes weren't expensive or fancy, but she had a way of making them look like they had just come out of a box just for her.

By 1994, Maureen's dad, G, was getting worse. He had struggled against lung cancer, and Maureen had been to visit him countless times, sometimes with the boys and sometimes on her own. We got a call one night that an aneurism had gone to his brain and killed him. Even though she knew it was coming, it hit her hard. He was her rock, her foundation, and now he was gone. I watched her at the funeral, watched her follow his casket to the graveside, and I thought how much like him she was. She kept her head high and gave him love and dignity in her good-bye. She told Erik and Ryan he would always be their grandfather, and he was still there for them in their hearts. She didn't let them see her break down. She kept her grief to herself and turned her face to the future and the family she had in our little house.

That Halloween Maureen made costumes for the boys that just about knocked me out. She used cardboard boxes and covered them with construction paper and big loops of bright-colored cloth. They looked like friendly dragons or cartoon robots. When the kids tried to walk, they bumped into everything because they couldn't see. We laughed pretty hard, and then Maureen told them to take their heads off so they could go trick or treating. Every holiday was a chance for her to celebrate.

Chapter Two

Community

It was now November, and I don't know if it was before or after Thanksgiving in 1994, but I remember Maureen calling me into our bedroom.

"Bill, feel this," she said. She was sitting with her bra off holding her left breast. She had her fingers on one spot, so I didn't have to go looking. I felt a hard spot.

"What is it?" I asked. I'm just Bill; I'm a landscaper.

"It's a lump or something."

"Well how long has it been there?"

"I just now felt it."

"How long do you think it's been there? A week?"

"At the most a week." Maureen always did self-breast exams. I know that for a fact. As a man you don't think of it, but Maureen knew to keep track of changes in her body.

"You had better get it checked out," I said.

"I know. I'm not fooling around with this."

The next day she made an appointment. "I want you to come with me."

It was the first time I saw uncertainty in her eyes. I said, "Sure, of course I'll go."

Maureen didn't want me to wait in the waiting room, she wanted me right there for the exam. When Doctor Peake came in, he looked a little surprised to see me. "Why are you here?" he asked Maureen.

She said, "We got a lump," and pointed to the area.

He started doing the examination, but he couldn't find it.

"Look, if you don't mind," said Maureen, "just let me have your hand and I'll put your fingers on the lump." She took his hand and placed it right where the lump was.

Dr. Peake nodded and agreed there was something there. "Can we agree that it's the size of a pea?"

Maureen nodded. "Yes, it feels a lot like a frozen pea."

"We'll schedule you for a mammogram, and we should probably do an ultra-sound as well."

It was then that Maureen said, "I saw a pamphlet in the waiting room that says the American Cancer Society will pay for mammograms. Can I do that?"

"Fine, if you want to call," was all that the doctor said. He didn't call for her or help out. It wasn't that we couldn't afford it, our health insurance paid for most of it, but Maureen was always very careful about money. She looked at the deductible and figured why not save the family a little money. It wasn't as if she wasn't going to follow through if they said no, but she believed it was her job to look after the family finances. That money was better spent on the boys or on something for the house. It was just her proving that every penny counts. She said, "When it comes to my health, I'm going to do the right thing, if I can save my family some money, I'm going to do that." The ACS paid for the mammo-gram but didn't pay for the Sonogram. Maureen had the Sonogram done just as Dr. Peake had recommended and paid for that herself.

I remember feeling like we were taking care of things. I didn't know then that Maureen feared cancer worse than anything else you could name.

Doctor Peake called Maureen after a few days with the results. "It's just calcifi-cation. The milk ducts get clogged sometimes," he said.

Questionable breast lump
Medical Record 11/9/94
C/0 lump left breast-noted 5 days ago.
Described by doctor as a 'pea-sized' moveable lesion on left breast. Draws it at the 5 o'clock position on the breast. Orders a mammogram.

"But I nursed my two babies," Maureen told him. "Why would my milk ducts be clogged?"

"Don't worry about it, it's no big deal. Just make sure you come back in next year for an annual mammogram. Cysts like this are common in women."

"Can this calcification turn into cancer?"

"No, absolutely not. Once it's calcification, it's always calcification."

Maureen called me at work right away. "Dr. Peake told me it was calcification of the milk ducts."

"You sound like you're still worried," I said. "What's bothering you?"

"I don't know. I just don't see why all of a sudden I have clogged milk ducts five years after nursing Ryan."

Further tests for breast lump
Medical Record 11/14/94
Asymmetric density in the inferior outer aspect of the left breast when compared to the right. In addition there are some small calcifications. Ultrasound recommended. The history indicates a palpable mass in that area. Following the ultrasound if there is no cyst, then biopsy recommended.

Medical Record 11/17/94
Two small cysts next to one another. These are responsible for the density seen on mammography. They measure approximately 1.7 cm total length.

I made a call to the doctor, because I didn't know anything about calcification or cysts. I asked him more questions about the lump. Maureen followed up her visit too with some phone calls to make sure she was O.K. Every time she was told it was nothing to worry about. It was great. It was wonderful. We heard everything we wanted to hear when we left the doctor's office. Life was back to normal after that first visit.

But life wasn't normal, because Maureen knew that she had this lump. I didn't know it bothered her so much. When she was eighteen or nineteen, she had a lump in her breast, and her mother took her right away to the doctors. It was a cyst. The doctor did a needle biopsy, and the cyst dissipated on its own. Maureen told me that at the time, she hadn't been worried. It seemed routine.

I thought everything was O.K. I held Maureen every night. For fifteen years I couldn't wait to get home. I got my hug in the kitchen and at night I held her. But Maureen was worried.

I didn't know it. Next morning was like every morning, much like at most people's house. Maureen woke up everyday with a grin and a spark in her eyes like, "O.K., it's another day!" If the boys didn't get up, she started hollering a little, nudging them along so they'd make the bus. She made them apple-cinnamon oatmeal, or she'd pour a bowl of *Frosted Mini-Wheats* and milk and put it in the microwave for Ryan. Erik liked cold cereal. On weekends, I made eggs or French toast. Maureen's dinners were nothing special, but she always had something hot and ready for the boys and me. She made meatloaf a lot, trying to stretch the dollars. Erik loved liver, so she cooked that up with onions. Ryan wouldn't touch it.

When Erik was nine and Ryan was seven, Maureen bought them b.b. guns. They had contests shooting at cans and got pretty good. Erik shot at a bird once. He didn't think he would hit it, but he did. He felt bad, because Maureen had told them the guns weren't for any living things, and she told them to never, ever shoot at cars. He never pointed his gun at anything but cans again.

When the boys got big enough to play sports, Maureen signed them up for soccer. She brought oranges for the whole team and stood on the sidelines, cheering and jumping when the team scored. The boys told her it was embarrassing, but she said she didn't care, it was a mom's right to cheer her kids on. One year the team didn't lose a game. She was right there patting all the kids on the back. If her boys got out of line, she spoke to them right then and there, whether it embarrassed them or not. She let them see it if she was mad, but she never swore.

A year or so later, Erik wanted to play the saxophone, so Maureen signed him up for that. He played the clarinet for a while too. Ryan took up the trumpet soon after, and Maureen and I went to all their school band concerts. She made sure they practiced right after their homework, and never did she let the boys speak disrespectfully. I came home from work one night and heard about Erik cursing in front of her. He was only trying to tell a joke, and I guess it had a curse word in it. They were in the car on the way to a friend's house and she almost didn't let him go. "That's not a word you're every going to use in this house," she told him. That was it.

Right about then, I was offered the job of grounds keeper and director of operations for a baseball facility built by the Chicago White Sox, called Sky Lands Park. The Cardinals own the ball field now. It was a good job, and I loved it, but when that operation went bankrupt, I went back to Steve Willands. All during this time, I was building up my own landscaping business, doing evening jobs in the summer or on weekends. Lots of folks in the development and all around Bushkill recognized how hard I worked.

Six months later, we were in our bedroom getting dressed for church and Maureen stopped as she was brushing her hair. I always liked watching her do her hair. She had the shiniest, thickest hair with big soft curls, and she made it look nice no matter where we were going. Even if we weren't going anywhere, she took the time to fix her hair. She looked at me in the mirror and said, "Bill, this lump is still bothering me."

I knew right away which lump she meant. "Why didn't you tell me?" I asked. I always wanted to know anything that upset her. Usually she let me know what was going on with her.

"Well, they said it was O.K. I didn't want to make a big deal out of it."

I watched her face as she talked, and I knew she had been brave for a while now. She turned to look at me directly, and I sat down on the bed.

"I know they said it wasn't anything to worry about, so why is it still bothering you?"

"I don't know. I just don't like this lump. It gets tender sometimes, and I can feel it."

It still doesn't dawn on me why she is so worried. We'd been to the doctor and he told us not to worry about it. But I took Maureen's worry seriously. "Call the doctor back," I said.

"I don't want to go to Doctor Peake," she said, and when she saw the question on my face, she added, "I know it might sound silly, but he's a man and he didn't really find the lump, I had to find it for him."

"Isn't there a woman doctor in the same network? Call her; go see her."

In May 1995, Maureen went to Doctor Berger six months after the test with Doctor Peake. Maureen brought up the fact that she had this lump and it was bothering her. She wanted this doctor's opinion. Doctor Berger felt her breast. I wasn't with her at this visit, because Maureen didn't want to make more out of it than it needed to be. She wouldn't have thought of me missing work if I didn't have to; she wanted everything to be normal. The lump just bothered her and she wanted a different opinion.

Growing concern over breast lump
Medical Record 5/3/95
Phone call from Maureen to Medical Group requesting an appointment.

Medical Record 5/4/95
"Patient states she still feels lump noted in November of 1994." Draws 2 palpable lumps at 3 and 6 o'clock. Recommends mammogram in November of 1995.

The doctor found the lump, and agreed at the size. She believed it was a little bigger than the first doctor had indicated, but she told Maureen she wasn't due for any tests for another year.

Routine doctor visit and more questions about breast lumps
Medical Record 10/4/95
Phone call from Maureen Thiel

Medical Record 10/14/95
Bronchitis

Medical Record 10/16/95
Purpose of visit is breast exam.
Doctor draws same palpable lumps at the 3 & 6 o'clock positions. Describes lumps as 'smooth, mobile and slightly tender, same as 5/95 exam.

The crazy thing is that Doctor Berger found another lump. The first one was still in the same place. It hadn't moved or changed for six months, and now there was another.

The doctor said, "You're not due for any more tests for another year." Maureen always followed doctor's orders, and she always asked lots of questions. But Maureen only waited six months before going back for another exam. Doctor Berger sent Maureen for another mammogram.

Breast lump assessment
Medical Record 10/26/95
Screening Mammogram: Since the study of 11/14/94 the left breast cysts have resolved. At this site within the inferomedial aspect of the left breast are noted numerous calcifications for which ancillary cone compression cc magnification & true lateral views of the breast would initially recommended in further accessing the number nature and distribution of these calcifications. There are no dominant masses.

Medical Record 10/27/95
Phone call from doctor to Maureen telling her that additional films are necessary.

Further mammograms
Medical Record 10/31/95
Diagnostic Mammography:
Included magnified compressed views and true lateral views. Area of calcifications in the inferior aspect of the left breast. The patient brought along films done in 1991 in Tampa, Florida, which revealed calcifications in that area at that time. These are believed to represent benign calcifications. Repeat study in one year recommended.

Diagnosis: Calcifications
Medical Record 11/1/95
Phone call from doctor to Maureen. Reports on mammogram as benign calcifications. Mammo to be repeated in 1 year.

The doctor called Maureen and told her she needed to have further mammogram films. These films magnified the area of her breast where the lump was located. Maureen was glad to have more information.

After the tests, Doctor Berger called and told Maureen she had benign calcifications. She said, "Come back in one year. Don't worry about it."

Maureen still had her lump, but she was optimistic. I was optimistic. She told me when I got home that everything was fine; cysts in the breast are pretty common. We were happy to hear what we heard. Life was still normal. I put the anxiety behind me, but I don't think Maureen ever did, and she knew she should go back in six months.

By early spring of 1996, the lumps were really bothering Maureen and now I knew it. When I held her tight at night, I always cuddled her with my arm over her breasts. That's the way we went to sleep every night. But she wouldn't let me hold her that way anymore. She told me her under wire bras made her breast sore too. I didn't know what to tell her.

Around that time Maureen had taken the boys to the pool and was sitting with the other moms while the kids splashed around. Maureen told me her lumps were under "open discussion" with the women. Patty Flotz told Maureen that she had had a breast lump, and that she had it removed. When Maureen told me, I could see how much she liked the idea.

"I can go to the doctor and get these lumps cut out and not worry about them any more," she said.

"Well, if it's nothing, let's do it."

Maureen went back to Doctor Berger and told her she wanted the lumps removed. But the doctor said, "You're not supposed to have more tests for six months."

Maureen insisted that she wanted to see a surgeon, so the doctor referred Maureen to a surgeon. Maureen just wanted to get the two lumps cut out. She had made her mind up and was ready to follow through. I went with her to the surgeon's office. I remember that visit well. Doctor Wald right away asked us, "What are you here for?"

Maureen brought with her every mammogram and ultrasound film that she'd had since Florida. He looked at a couple of the records. I don't even know if he looked at them all. I don't think he did. As we sat in his office, the doctor told us he was going to do another ultrasound on Maureen right away. He had an ultrasound machine in a room off his office and he called in a technician to do the ultrasound.

Referral to surgeon to assess breast lumps
Medical Record 5/10/96
C/o lumps in breast:
electrical charges/sensations especially with pressure from bra in left axilla.
Referral made to surgeon on this date.
Palpable nodules drawn at the 3 o'clock and 6 o'clock positions on the left breast.

Maureen was still in the surgical gown, and I was standing next to her with the technician when Doctor Wald came back into the room. He stood across from us and looked from one to the other. "I can't remove the two lumps."

Maureen almost jumped off the table. I think we both said, "Why?" at the same time.

"You have way too many lumps now. If we remove the two larger lumps, we would also have to remove part of your breast because of all the surrounding cysts."

Maureen's face went white and her fingers dug into my arm. I don't think either one of us was breathing. All Maureen's buried worries now surfaced like a geyser erupting.

"What do you mean I've got more lumps? I've been to the doctor every six months having mammograms and Sonagrams. I've done everything I've been told to do. I've even tried to go home and not worry. I was told not to worry, so I worked real hard at that. Now you're telling me my breast is full of lumps, not just one or two?" Her voice shook and cracked as it rose.

Doctor Wald looked down at Maureen and gave her a gentle smile. "Mrs. Thiel, I know this is difficult." He said it as if Maureen would have a hard time understanding. "You have fibrocystic disease. Many women have this and live with it all their lives. Get dressed and meet me at the reception counter."

Breast lumps noted; diagnosed as cysts
Medical Record 5/14/96
In a letter to primary care doctor,
surgeon notes 3 discrete areas in the left breast:
4 o'clock, 6 o'clock and 9 o'clock positions.
These are distinct from the remainder of the breast tissue.
There is nothing to suggest by palpation that these are suspicious for malignancy.
The axilla are negative.
Repeat ultrasound in 6 months to see if cysts are changing.
If any changes are noted aspiration may be indicated.

Medical Record 5/14/96
Ultrasound: Multiple cysts are noted throughout the left breast.
These appear to be simple cysts compatible with fibrocystic disease.

Maureen was shaking and trying real hard not to cry. I helped her get the gown off and she pulled on her bra and shirt. Her hands fumbled at the buttons, but she shook her head when I tried to help. She tried to get hold of herself. We left all the films on the surgeon's desk and went out to the reception area. The doctor came out and put his arm around her. "Maureen, this is common," he said.

I stood right there, and Maureen tried to calm down. I tried to calm her down. She took big gulps of air and kept smoothing her hair and wiping at her eyes. She looked at me and then looked up at the surgeon, her eyes huge, "I'm so afraid of cancer."

I'll never forget her saying that.

"I can assure you, you don't have cancer." Those were Doctor Wald's exact words. I based everything on those words after we left. I leaned on those words in the way I lived with Maureen and loved her and tried to keep her mind away from her fears.

"Maureen," the surgeon added, "we'll keep an eye on this fibrocystic disease. It's very common and it's not cancer. Come back in six months."

We were still standing at the counter and Maureen turned to the receptionist. "I need to make an appointment. When should I make it?"

"Don't call us, we'll call you," Doctor Wald said then he turned to the receptionist. "I assured Maureen that we're going to watch this for her."

That comforted Maureen and it helped me too. He didn't give us the cancer word. We could live with it.

I was glad and eventually Maureen was glad. We were just going to have to live with these lumps. Maureen rebounded, and everything was the same except I couldn't hold her the same way. I put my arm around her waist instead. That's no big deal. We settled back into our everyday selves, getting the kids up for school, walking the dogs, having barbecues, talking about summer camping trips. Maureen never let me know how much those lumps still bothered her. Neither one of us gave it much thought at the time, but because of my work, we had a new health insurance company, which meant we had to find new doctors. I always let Maureen handle that part.

New Health Insurance
Medical Record 7/96
Insurance changed to U.S. Healthcare

In 1996 Maureen got the idea to organize a trip to Knoebles Amusement Park and then Promise Land for camping. Eleven to thirteen families came. We spent the whole day going on rides then at night we camped out. We cooked over the fire or bought hot dogs and ice cream cones at a stand across from the campground. Every family had their own site, but we cooked and ate together and then sat around the fire talking. No one cared what anybody looked like in the morning. Maureen, who always had her make up and hair just right, didn't care either up at the park. Sometimes we sat up all night talking. That campout became the Maureen Thiel Annual Campout for the families. All the Promise Land rangers needed to hear was the name, 'Maureen Thiel' and they would help out, because we were such regulars. I think Patty and Rob Flotz and a few other families still go.

When we weren't out on longer trips, we biked around the area or went rollerblading. I never did like ice skating or being cold. One of our favorite bike rides was down Brisco Mountain Road. It's a small, curved road that cuts through acres of wild rhododendrons, witch hazel, white pines and sugar maples. We packed a lunch and rode around for hours. I drove down that road one early spring day and saw a black bear at the side of the road. I stopped and rolled down my window. I could smell him, and he smelled like bear.

Through all those days, Maureen still had her gut feeling, but when she had been told by so many people that she was wrong, she began to believe that maybe she was. It was hard for her, but after we left the surgeon's office, she said, "Bill, maybe I have been worrying too much. Maybe I have been a little crazy about cancer and making too much of this. I'm going to stop pushing. That's it, we're going on vacation and we're going to forget about this and not worry. We're putting this behind us."

Routine doctor visit
Medical Record 9/20/96
Office Visit to new primary care physician Chief complaint is problem with the throat. No breast exam or breast complaints noted in this visit.

We made a trip to Disney World, Florida in the fall of 1996. It wasn't exactly a second honeymoon, because we had the boys with us, but we visited all the places we liked to go when we lived down there. I didn't need another honeymoon. I was glad to open my eyes every morning and find Maureen beside me. The boys had a great time, and Maureen was so happy taking them all around.

We had a wonderful Christmas and New Years that winter too. Maureen decorated our house like it was Santa's own house. Because of the way we put up lights on the house, we were written up in the local papers and folks would stop by and take pictures. It was Christmas land, and Maureen was the elf who made every one feel like a kid getting a present.

Right about this time, I was ready to leave Steve Willand for the second time, because my landscape business was going well. I figured the business was ready to take off, and March would be the perfect time to launch out on my own again. In late February of 1997, I was in the living room measuring a corner for a set of shelves when I heard Maureen call.

"Bill, come here." I didn't like the familiar sound of those words or the tone of her voice.

"What's wrong?"

"Can you feel this?" She was sitting on the edge of the bed, just where she had been the first time. She had come out of the shower, so she had a towel wrapped around her body and another one turban-like around her hair. I felt under her arm.

"What is that?" I knew, but I didn't want to know.

"A lump."

"Damn it, Maureen!"

We just looked at each other for a few seconds and I saw the fear rising. I said quickly, "Well, it's not near your breast, that's a good thing." I had no clue what a lump was doing under her arm.

"I'm calling the doctor," she said, her voice tight. She didn't even take the time to get dressed, just hitched the towel around her and went for the phone. Our health insurance had changed since Maureen had last been to the primary care doctor. We had a new family physician and she asked him about a gynecologist she could see for pap smears and these lumps.

The day of the appointment was blustery and there were dark clouds coming in from the west. By early afternoon we were in the middle of a snow storm and the schools were closing early. Maureen stood at the living room window, chewing her lip, looking out at the roads.

"I don't know, Bill. Maybe I should reschedule." She was more talking out loud than asking me. She started for the phone, then stopped, looked out the window again, and said, "No, I'm going. I don't want to wait any more."

A new lump
Medical Record 3/3/97
c/c increasing lump breast. Nurse documents complaint of lump under left arm. Dr. notes firm nodule in the left breast and draws it at the 6 o'clock position. Makes referral for a mammogram and surgical consult.

Medical Record 3/6/97
"Suspicious density 6 o'clock position of left breast with overlying calcifications. There are prominent left axillary lymph nodes not clearly appreciated on the previous mammogram of 10/25/95.
Sonography will be done for additional evaluation.

Medical Record 3/6/97
Ultrasound Left Breast: "Complex mass in 6 o'clock position. Biopsy is recommended to rule out possible malignancy.

The roads were awful. Twice the car fishtailed as we went round a curve, but I never suggested going back. Everything in Maureen was pointed for that doctor's office. When we got to the appointment and into the exam room, Maureen explained to Doctor Jackson about the lumps and everything she had been told. She told him about all the mammograms and ultrasounds then she pointed to the new lump under her arm. The doctor felt all the lumps. He scheduled her for a mammogram and ultrasound right away.

We went back to hear the results of the tests. Doctor Jackson didn't waste time. "I want you to make an appointment with a surgeon."

After what we had heard from every other doctor, we both looked at him startled. "What do you mean?" asked Maureen.

"I want to get this lump out," he said. "I want to do a biopsy." It was the first time we heard the word biopsy. "I'll refer you to a good surgeon."

Doctor Jackson sent us to a surgeon, Doctor Schuster, and we scheduled the biopsy for the next week. That was the soonest he could do it. Maureen would have had them do it right then if she could have.

Maureen's worries surfaced again; she was so anxious, just worried to death. I only wanted to get her through the appointment with the surgeon. The faster I could get her there, the faster he could get the lump out, and then we'd be back to normal. That's what I thought would happen. We wouldn't have to worry about cancer or cysts. All those doctors had said, "Don't worry."

We were to meet the surgeon at the same-day surgery. Easy, you know, just in and out. That morning before we went, I asked Maureen how she was doing.

"I'm O.K," she said.

But she had been restless all night, and now she seemed excited, like her nerves had twisted her worry around to look forward and hope everything was finally going to be over. "It's no big deal, just a lump removal," she added. "We'll probably be home by noon and you can go back to work."

Biopsy recommended
Medical Record 3/11/97
Office Visit with Surgeon
3-4 cm mobile mass left breast @ 6 o' clock recommends excisional biopsy

---

Of course she was nervous, but she managed to keep going. Maureen never got stuck in fear or feeling sorry. She could have a leg cut off, and the next day she'd be on two crutches and trying to figure out a way to go forward. She wouldn't sit and whine. That's just the way she was made.

On March 18, 1997, we headed over Dingman's Bridge for Newton Memorial Hospital for same-day surgery.

Chapter Three

The Scream

That morning we drove out of the neighborhood and got on Route 209, my usual way to work. After crossing Dingmans Bridge we rode along the Delaware River for a few miles until we picked up Rte 206 in New Jersey at the intersection where the Layton General Store stands. The General store is a red clapboard, one-story affair with a wide wooden porch no more than a step from the road. A few years back they had to take out a window and use a crane to get a hunter's world-record, 900-lb. black bear inside. That store marks the turn that pointed us directly toward Newton. As we drove, the land leveled and the terrain opened into farm fields with horse paddocks and gambrel-roofed barns. The forest had been cut down for crops and now makes room for the occasional strip mall and small industrial park. We passed Owassa and Culver Lakes with their camp-grounds, we passed our dentist, and further down the road the New Jersey State Fair Grounds and Steve Willand's equipment business where I worked. Another ten minutes and we arrived at Newton Memorial Hospital. Built in the late 1800s, the original hospital is an old red brick building, classic, the kind of building they made for town halls, schools and hospitals.

As we moved down the hallways, the resort-like mauves and peaches gave way to blue and gray hospital linoleum, beige and blue curtains over outpatient nooks and the Formica tops of the nurses' stations. Monitors, wheelchairs, clipboards, red plastic bins for toxic substance disposal and the sound of rubber-soled hospital staff surrounded us. Maureen had my hand so tight I could feel each of her fingers leaving a dent. I just let her hold on.

I brought Maureen into the same-day surgery area and we filled out all of the forms they always have. A nurse came and told Maureen to follow her to a room where she could change from her clothes to a hospital gown. Before they left, the nurse pointed to the waiting area and said, "Make yourself comfortable, Mr. Thiel. We'll come and get you when your wife is in the recovery room."

I kissed Maureen on her forehead. "You're going to be fine," I told her. She looked at me and nodded, then she turned and I watched her walk down the hall next to the nurse. I found out later they had to sedate Maureen almost as soon as they got her in the room, because she couldn't stop crying. I guess she started crying as soon as I was out of earshot.

I took a seat in the waiting room and then stood up again to get a cup of coffee. The chairs in the waiting area had probably started out being in straight lines, but with people coming and going, and some people needing to put their feet up or pull closer to whoever brought them, the chairs had become clumped and uneven. Like everyone else, I was sitting there with people I'd met for the first time. We were all in the waiting room, and each of us had somebody in there having their same-day procedure. I was waiting for Maureen, my wife.

I smiled at an old man who was going through the motions of turning the pages of a magazine. I sat back down and sipped my coffee. He asked me what I was there for and I told him. He was waiting for his wife too, he said. She was having a mole removed from her leg. He told me the whole story of her moles and then we got on to where they lived and how many grandkids they had. He was quite a talker, I remember that. We chatted for a long time and then his wife appeared and they left. I sat watching the nurses and orderlies coming and going and I saw a woman bring in a little girl with her hand all wrapped up in a dish cloth. The girl's face was blotchy from crying and the mom's lips were pressed in a thin hard line.

And then I heard a scream. The scream engulfed everything. It lashed down the hall like an electric charge. It filled each space it found and jolted every nerve. We all turned to it. We couldn't help it. The scream controlled us as it rose and expanded into layers of screams. It was the scream you'd make if your hand was cut off. The scream you'd make if your child was run over. The scream of being raped. The scream of going over a cliff. I looked for the ambulance, for the flashing lights, for the stretcher all bloody. I looked for the emergency room. But the scream came toward me and it was calling my name.

I could hear Maureen screaming in fear and anger. That scream split our life in two. It split one moment from the next, split the life we knew from the life we would now have. All I could hear was the scream. It was fearful, and everything happened in seconds. I saw the gurney with nurses running and pushing it. The scream was coming from the gurney. Maureen was the scream. The doctor was a few feet in front, and he had his eye focused on me. The scream pinned my heart to the floor. It's been eight years and I haven't stopped hearing that scream yet.

As soon as Maureen saw me, she yelled, "Bill! Bill! It's cancer, Bill!" Those were her first words. Then she yelled, as mad as I've ever heard anyone, "I'm going to sue those fucking doctors!" Maureen never got mad and she never, ever swore.

All I heard was 'cancer'. I heard other things, but they weren't anything that made sense. One plus one didn't equal two. She was still being rolled down the hallway, fifteen, twenty feet to the recovery room and they were injecting her with tranquilizers. The doctor grabbed my arm and pulled me into a little room off the hallway. My heart was beating four thousand miles an hour. He sat me down and said, "Bill, it's bad."

Before the scream we should have had a warning. Maureen did all the right things. She asked all the right questions. But when someone else is making the decisions, sometimes the right questions don't matter, especially if you get the wrong answers. We didn't know they were the wrong answers; we were trying to make our lives the best we could.

It took a long time before the tranquilizer took hold and Maureen quieted down. The surgeon tried to talk to me in another room, but all I could hear was 'cancer'.

Maureen had cancer now. Her biggest fear. There were a million things that I'll never know that probably went through her mind. My mind raced all over the place and I was so afraid. There is no monster I can think of that could make me that scared. The pathology report stated that the lump Maureen had first found in November of 1994, was cancerous. It also stated that the cancer had spread into the milk ducts and into the lymph node that they removed from under her arm.

Biopsy performed and diagnosed
Medical Record 3/18/97
Excisional Biopsy left Breast Mass:
Mass described as 3 cm at 6 o'clock position Path report: Infiltrating intraductal carcinoma poorly differentiated grade III size 3.5 x 2.5 x 2.5. Angiolymphatic invasion present.

After the pathology report came back, the oncology surgeon wanted to look at more of Maureen's lymph nodes. Neither our regular doctor nor the surgeon wanted to waste any time. Maureen had enough time to get home and recuperate a little from the first surgery. None of us told her how bad things looked. We didn't tell the boys anything. I thought, and I think Maureen thought too, that maybe there would be a different story after the second surgery. Maybe the surgeon would find out something different. We were right about a different story. It just wasn't the story we wanted to hear. Right away, a week later, in she went again. We had to go back; the surgeon had scraped and he wanted to take more. That's all I remember. He said he didn't feel like he got enough.

I went in to see Maureen after the second surgery. She was wrung out.

"It hurts, Bill," was the first thing she said. No big smile to let me know she was all right. I asked her where and how bad.

"All under my arm and down my side," she told me. "It feels like they tore out bunches of grapes."

What she felt was lymph nodes being removed. She was in the hospital for three days. The lab dissected all those lymph nodes. Doctor Schuster said, "Bill, I removed 47 lymph nodes from your wife and the pathology report has come back; every one of them is positive." I didn't understand what he meant; I knew nothing about lymph nodes. I probably asked him many questions I'll never remember. I remember him telling me, because I must have asked the question: "Is this curable, or how long do I get her, how many years do I have with her?" He flat told me she probably wasn't going to live two years.

Lymph nodes removed, sent to lab
Medical Record 3/26/97
Re-excision of biopsy site left breast with left axillary node dissection.
Path report: 47 nodes resected-47 nodes positive for metastatic poorly differentiated ductal carcinoma gr III.

Medical Record 3/27/97
CT abdomen and chest read as normal.

Medical Record 3/28/97
Whole Body Bone Scan: "negative study"

You know when a leaf gets so dry it just crumbles when you touch it, just falls away into dust? That's how my insides felt. Like everything living inside had just been turned to dust.

By removing the lymph nodes, the doctor and the laboratory found that Maureen had Stage III breast cancer. I had to learn fast. It was like no other lesson I ever learned. There are five basic stages to breast cancer. The first is Stage 0 or "in situ," which means "in place". That means the cancer is contained and hasn't spread. The American Cancer Society says the survival rate for women with Stage 0 is 100%. Stage I is when the cancer is only about 2 centimeters or ¾ of an inch and hasn't spread to any lymph nodes. If a woman lives for five years after being diagnosed with this stage of cancer, her chances of survival are about 98%.

Stage IIA means the cancer is between 2 and 5 centimeters and still hasn't gone into any lymph nodes: her chance of survival after five years are about 88%. Stage IIB means the cancer is still about the same size, but it has moved into the lymph nodes under the arm; chances of survival are about 76%.

When the cancer is still around 2 to 5 centimeters but has moved into the underarm lymph nodes and underarm tissue, that's Stage IIIA; chances of survival are about 56%. If the cancer is of any size, or has attached itself to the chest wall and spread to the chest lymph nodes as well as the armpit lymph nodes and tissue, then it's Stage IIIB. Maureen had Stage IIIB. Her chance of making it through this, according to the American Cancer Society was about 49%. Less then a toss of a coin. The cancer had spread to all the lymph nodes under her arm and in her chest.

Those are all the stages, but at that moment I didn't know anything about lymph nodes. So I read. Lymph nodes are like little pods or beads strung along a web that runs through the whole body. Most of them are in the armpit area, neck, the abdomen and the groin. Everyone has a different number of lymph nodes, but the average number in the armpit area is 15 to 30. Maureen had 47 lymph nodes removed, which meant they took out all of them in her armpit, down her arm and in the left side of her chest. Every single one of them had cancer in them, because that's what lymph nodes do.

Lymph nodes are made of special tissue to help fight infections and diseases like cancer. They reproduce to help when things are going really bad, until, like in any battle, they are overwhelmed and can't keep fighting. The Stage III part meant the cancer had spread not only to the lymph nodes under her arm which are the axillary lymph nodes, but into more breast and arm tissue also. I found this out later. Doctor Schuster told me that he couldn't operate on her breast, because the tumor was too widespread. He wanted to use chemotherapy to shrink it before he operated.

In the hospital, Maureen did finally settle down. I don't know what I said to get in to see her. If they had told me I had to chew through iron or claw my way through concrete to get to her, it wouldn't have mattered. I had to be with her. They drugged her pretty good because she was in recovery for hours.

I wasn't settled down. I had lived with days of crying after we found out she had cancer. They told me she was going to live less than two years. I couldn't tell her that. That evening when Maureen came out of recovery, she was ready to fight. She thought the doctor had told her he had removed four to seven lymph nodes, not 47 malignant nodes. I wasn't going to argue with her. I even thought maybe I had misunderstood the doctor. Maureen had the drains hanging out of her arm from the lymph node dissection, but she was ready to beat the cancer.

Maureen was in a semi-private room, sharing it with a woman who had liver cancer. I remember the woman being wheeled back into the room after they had done a second stomach tap. Her doctor came in and closed the curtain. He told her to go home and get her affairs together. There couldn't be another tap. I thought, "That's not going to be us."

The afternoon I brought Maureen home, I pulled up in front of the house, and came around and opened Maureen's door, but she just sat there.

"I can't Bill." Tears poured down her face. "I can't look at the boys right now. I don't want them to see me crying and with all these tubes hanging out."

I crouched down next to her and she put her head on my shoulder. "It's O.K., Maureen. Take as long as you want. Erik knows; I told him yesterday when he came home from his ski trip. Ryan doesn't know yet."

Tears came hard again then she sat up and wiped her face. "I don't have time to sit here and cry, Bill. Help me out."

She was just out of the car when the boys came out of the house. They came toward her, not sure, both their eyes huge, looking at their mom to see if she was all right. Maureen grabbed them both. She went down on her knees and hugged them like it was the last hug she was ever going to get, like she had never held them before. She wrapped her arms around them, and she was practically choking them because she was afraid to let them go.

Erik and Ryan had never seen her so scared and upset. They held her too and tried to understand. Erik was eleven and Ryan was nine. It was the first day of a new life, and now Maureen's biggest fear had become real. She had her two kids right in front of her, right in her arms. That was her focus from then on, her two kids. When her fear got the worst of her, she closed her eyes and put herself there with her two kids. They were everything. Her fight, her desire, her will to live, everything revolved around Erik and Ryan.

The next day she sat Ryan down after school and told him she was very sick. I watched from the kitchen, watched her hug him and try to explain. She cried; she couldn't help it. Ryan was confused, he couldn't imagine his mom afraid of anything or that anything bad could happen to her.

Less than seven days after Maureen had the second surgery, I came home from work and found strange cars in the driveway. I remember thinking to myself, "What's going on?" I thought it was the police in unmarked cars. I parked in a hurry and went in the house to find people in suits with cameras and video recorders. Maureen sat on the couch, looking almost like she always did when we had company.

"Bill," she said, "I want you to meet Mr. MacDonald, and Mr. McGregor and this is Marcia Kohanski."

I know I said "Hello, pleased to meet you," or something like that, but I turned to Maureen bewildered. "Who are they?"

"They're lawyers."

With 47 lymph nodes just removed and the tubes still in, Maureen had driven to Stroudsburg to see these lawyers. With no hard evidence, just the story Maureen told, the Foley law firm took her case. Michael and Malcolm are lawyers and Marcia is a nurse who works with the firm.

"Mr. Thiel," said Michael MacDonald, "your wife has a hell of a story. She has a serious issue here."

I knew how angry she was about the doctors, and I knew what she had screamed when she came out of surgery, but I had no idea what she was doing.

"What's going on?" I asked.

"She's filing a law suit against the three doctors that she saw before this surgery," answered Malcolm McGregor.

I couldn't make sense of it.

"She's suing the doctors."

All I could say was "O.K." I cared what Maureen was doing, but I couldn't take it all in. I understood how mad Maureen was, but there were lawyers in my house only a week after her surgery. Maureen had not even begun to heal, but while I was at work, Maureen had driven eighteen miles over mountain roads with the boys to Stroudsburg to meet these lawyers and tell them what had happened. Now she sat on our living room couch ready to make sure the doctors didn't get away with anything.

I just sat and listened. Malcolm could tell I was bewildered so he explained. "When Maureen came to the office, we knew pretty quickly that she had a case. She told us, 'I've had this lump in my breast forever. And I was telling them and telling them.' She brought her records with her, so she knows she is in big trouble, but she has hope. She had the boys with her, and they colored with markers while we talked. She told us how she knew in her heart something was wrong, she kept telling the doctors. None of this is her fault."

At that point Maureen exploded again. "I'm so angry! How can they get away with this? What if this happens to someone else? Do other women know this can happen to them? I told the doctors, I kept pointing to it. There's a lump in my breast, and they told me it was nothing. And now they tell me it's cancer all through my lymph nodes, and I have to go through all this therapy." Maureen's anger filled the room, but she wasn't crying. She was going to make the doctors own up to what they had said and done and make sure it didn't happen again. Maureen and the lawyers talked for a while. Maureen especially talked to Marcia.

I think Marcia was one of the reasons Maureen liked the Foley Law Firm at the beginning. Marcia was easy for Maureen to talk with and she understood what Maureen was trying to do.

At one point either Michael or Malcolm said, "There's no guarantee you'll get any financial settlement from this case, Mrs. Thiel. We want to be clear about that. The majority of malpractice suits don't result in large awards or even in any award."

Maureen looked directly at him and said, "I never want this to happen to another woman. And I want to help my boys. I want my family to be O.K. That's all I want." She said it in an even, clear voice. End of discussion.

After they left, Maureen talked about how furious she was and she didn't understand how the doctors did and said what they did. "I don't want this to ever happen to anyone else." It was in one ear and out the other to me. I focused on learning about cancer. I never even thought about the lawyers much after March of 1997. We saw them a few times over the next few months, but I never thought about the lawyers. It was important to me to be with Maureen. When it was important for Maureen to see the lawyers, then it was important to me. At that point, my job was saving her life. I let everything else go and put all my mind and heart on taking care of Maureen.

After the surgeries and after the visit from the lawyers, we moved right into the oncology phase. Maureen was totally destroyed, and I don't know how many days she cried. I was destroyed too. The surgeon told me that Maureen was probably not going to live two more years. How did he know that? I don't know. Neither the doctors nor I ever told her. When I knew I was right about the forty-seven positive lymph nodes, I never told her that either. I had a good reason. Maureen had to fight like hell. She didn't have many chances. God was calling, and I wasn't ready to give her up. I didn't want to fight God over her, but I did. The only thing that was relevant was Maureen and the cancer. Anyone would do the same. I put blinders on and focused on the cancer and my wife, that's what I did. I was going to lose my wife, my best friend. I thanked God every day for her. But I had so many questions.

I realized I'd better start learning. I did what anybody would do. I educated myself. I was just like lots of other husbands, reading so much you're eyes go bad and you have to get glasses, and if you don't, you didn't read enough. And if you have glasses already, you're probably going to need stronger ones after all the reading.

I got piles of information, lists of phone numbers, and Maureen got information too. We had two little computers that we filled with everything we could find. I called The American Cancer Society, and they tried to answer every question I asked them. I did not make these phone calls around Maureen, because not all the questions or answers were positive. I was ready to fight, don't get me wrong, but I had to educate myself in a different way than Maureen. I was asking different questions.

The American Cancer Society told me that they would put me in touch with people who were going through the same thing as Maureen. I asked them to have somebody call me that had 47 positive lymph nodes. I waited, and I called them again. I said, "You were going to have somebody call me that had 47 positive lymph nodes." There wasn't very much conversation after that. The people on the help line couldn't find anyone alive that had 47 positive lymph nodes. When the doctor told me it was bad, that's what he meant.

One day not long after the surgery and the lawyers, I told her I wasn't going to work. We had an appointment at one and I wanted to be there.

"No, Bill," Maureen said, "you go on. This is only a follow up after the surgery to check the stitches and the drains. I'll be all right."

In my heart I was saying, "Oh my God, this woman!" This woman isn't going to last two years unless God doesn't need her. That's what I told myself. That's the way I think. God says when he needs us. Both Maureen and I knew that when the Lord called us it would be an honor, but I wasn't ready for him to call her. I couldn't tell her what I was thinking. I went to work.

A week later, we went back to the doctors and had our first meeting with the oncologist, Doctor Mullen. Maureen had zillions of questions. Doctor Mullen told her she would have a round of chemotherapy, followed by more surgery, followed by radiation. Maureen just wanted to fight. She said, "Just tell me what I have to do. Let's go. Let's go fight this thing." Right away she wanted to know what the plan was. She never asked, "Can I beat this?" She just said "I'm going beat it. Tell me what we're going do." That was all I could think of myself.

Doctor Mullen was there from that day on, and Maureen started chemotherapy in April of 1997. She still had her breast and she was optimistic. She kept me going forward even though I was dying inside.

Oncologist recommends chemotherapy
Medical Record 3/31/97
Family History: father lung Ca; Grandmother some form of Ca
Oncologist stages the cancer a T2 N1
Suggests high dose Adriamycin & Cytoxan followed by radiation.

The oncologist told us exactly what was going on with the tumor before Maureen started on the chemotherapy. T2 meant the size of the tumor—it was between 2 and 5 centimeters in diameter. N1 meant the cancer had spread to the lymph nodes on the same side of her body as the breast that had the tumor. Doctor Mullen told us that after the chemotherapy, Maureen would have a mastectomy followed by radiation. From then on we went to the doctors every week, sometimes it was every day. During one of the visits, Doctor Mullen felt more swollen lymph nodes in her chest.

Adriamycin is the common name of Doxorubicin Hydrochloride, and it's a powerful drug that the doctors injected into Maureen. The largest dose you can get is 75 mg. That's what Maureen got. They told us this drug is used successfully to 'produce regression in breast carcinoma'. That's what we wanted to hear. They also told us that with high doses there is a risk of congestive heart failure. We put our hopes on 'regression'.

Cancer is aggressive
Medical Record 4/4/97
2 supraclavicular lymph nodes palpable

Chemotherapy begins
Medical Record 4/8/97
First cycle Adriamycin & Cytoxan

Maureen also had to take Cytoxan which is really cyclophophamide, another drug that combats cancer. This was the one that really made Maureen throw up even though they gave her something to help make her feel less nauseous. The Cytoxan also slowed her bone marrow from making white blood cells which fight against infection and make platelets to help prevent bleeding. Besides all that, they told us it would cause alopecia or hair loss and maybe irritate Maureen's bladder. She had to drink three quarts of water every day for three days after each dose. She did everything they told her to do. The amount of drugs they gave her made it hard for them to give it to her in regular shots. Instead of putting it into a little vein in her arm like driving on a back road, they wanted a direct route like a main highway, right into her chest.

Shunt inserted
Medical Record 4/15/97
Dr. suggests insertion of Porta-cath

Medical Record 4/21/97
Insertion of right subclavian porta-cath

To gain access for the drugs, they made an opening in one of her chest veins and put a little valve on it with a closeable seal. It meant she would have a plastic tube attached to her vein and have a small plastic valve hanging out of her chest. If that made things easier, that was all right with Maureen. It also meant we had to follow strict orders to keep it clean and dry. If any dirt or dampness got in there, Maureen could get an infection and that would mean more drugs and slow up the chemotherapy. We were more than careful. It became my job to wrap her up before she took a shower and to clean out the porta-cath every time it needed to be accessed. I wasn't taking any chances. I took off days from work, and went to every doctor's visit and chemotherapy session. I forgot about everything else; I had to try and save her.

Radiation Oncologist Assessment
Medical Record 4/25/97
Radiation Oncologist
Stages Cancer as T2 N1b M1 ER/PR negative

Maureen and I just listened to the doctors and made our decisions, but even that was hard. Maureen wanted to get as many doctor's opinions as she could. We read everything and asked as many questions as we could think of. She knew radiation was one treatment for cancer so we went to see a radiation oncologist. He became part of the team too.

After two chemotherapy treatments the tumor was still a T2 or between 2 and 5 centimeters. The N1b meant it was still present in the lymph nodes and tissue in her chest. The M1 meant Maureen had moved from Stage III cancer to Stage IV. Stage IV is the last stage. They treat it by thinking about survival time and relieving symptoms. ER/PR negative meant that Maureen had little or no estrogen or progesterone in her breast tissue. These two hormones are important to have, because they help fight cancer and bring on a remission. Maureen was out of luck there.

But Maureen was a fighter. No matter how bad I was dying inside, she wouldn't know it, because I wouldn't let her know it. I hid it as best I could, even at work. One day I snuck behind the building where I was working and got between the wooden pallets that were stacked in rows 30 and 40 high. I would squeeze behind them and sit in that quiet space. One day Steve Willand found me back there crying. He sent me home, saying, "Bill get out of here, go be with your wife." I had no words, I couldn't even stop crying. I got in my car and went home. I didn't say "Thank you," or even "O.K. I'm sorry, I'll get better". There were no words. I got home where I belonged. I just couldn't stop crying.

The doctors told Maureen she was going to lose all her beautiful, thick dark hair. They said it would probably come back. All her life, Maureen never wanted to do anything but make other people's hair beautiful.

Chemotherapy continues
Medical Record 5/1/97
Second cycle Adriamycin & Cytoxan

Medical Record 5/22/97
Third cycle of Adriamycin & Cytoxan

She was a beautiful hairdresser, and her hair was perfect all the time. Everywhere she went, everyone commented about her hair, everyone knew she was a hairdresser. Now she wasn't going to have any hair. But it would come back. She could live with that, and she was fighting with the chemotherapy. Every day when we had to go for the chemo she said, "Let's go, I'm gonna beat this."

But it was a big deal that she was going to lose her hair. They told us that maybe it wouldn't come out, but if it did, it was going to come out in little bits and more little bits and then it was going to come out in clumps.

Maureen came out of the shower crying one morning and I asked her what was wrong.

"It hurts, Bill. It just hurts to see all my hair clogging up the drain."

I took her in my arms and held her.

"I try to tell myself that it's the chemo working." She tried to smile through the tears running down her face. "If it's making my hair fall out, then it's killing the cancer cells too. But I feel so lost when I see all that hair. It makes me all shaky inside."

"Shhh, it's O.K.," I whispered. "It's O.K. to be scared." It wasn't just the shower drain. I'd find small clumps on her pillow or on the back of the couch where she'd been sitting. I knew she saw them too. It bothered her to see her hair lying there. It was one more thing to try to accept.

She leaned back and looked up at me. "I want you to shave my head."

I didn't say anything, just looked at her and saw how serious she was. She didn't want to see her hair falling out any more. Maureen went down to her salon and cut her hair real short. I took a picture of her like that and then we went into the bathroom. Her tears had stopped and she didn't say a word. I went very slowly and gently.

"It feels better," she said when I was done, but she didn't spend much time looking in the mirror. I took her by the hand and led her out to the couch.

"Sit here for a minute, I'll be right back." I went back into the bathroom and shaved my own head. I don't know exactly why, I just thought maybe it'd help her if we looked the same. When I came out of the bathroom, she burst out laughing.

"Oh, Bill! You look awful!"

I put my head down next to hers and we rubbed them together. We were both laughing. I knew I was funny looking enough without shaving my head. Then I took her hand and rubbed it over my head and that made her laugh again. It was worth it to hear that wonderful laugh.

"We must look like quite a pair!" She kept giggling as I showed her the back of my head.

I think it helped the boys see the change in their mom to have me change too, like it was an ordinary thing. Shortly after Maureen and I shaved our heads, the word went out. There was a parade of men in our house. All of Erik's and Ryan's friends and their fathers, all of Maureen's friends' husbands, and my friends came and had Maureen shave their head. She had no energy because of the chemo, but she shaved every one of them. Those friends did more for Maureen's hope and spirits than any drug. I still do not have enough thank yous for all those good people. I wish I could tell them what they did for Maureen that day. More than they knew. She tried to tell them, but I think it was hard for them to grasp the whole thing. We saw and felt the caring they had for her and I'll never forget it.

It was a wonderful gesture of all that Maureen meant to them. All the women, Maureen's friends Patty, Laurie, Helen, looked at Maureen and saw themselves sitting there. I'm sure they were scared, but they brought us so much joy.

After her hair was really gone, Maureen got wigs from the American Cancer Society. She made those wigs look just like her own hair. I couldn't believe what she could do with them, no one could believe it. We all joked with her about how skilled she was with the wigs. We all tried to get Maureen to laugh during those months. And most of the time it wasn't too hard. She laughed pretty easily. I came home from work on day and there was a strange woman in my kitchen. She turned around and winked.

"Hey, Bill," she said, "Fancy a blond tonight?"

Maureen caught me so by surprise, I think I even turned red. That made her laugh real hard and say, "It's O.K., Bill. I figured you deserved a treat."

She surprised the boys with the blond one too. Ryan didn't recognize her at all and kept smiling at her like she was some lady come to visit. Erik just kept laughing. She let the boys try on the wigs. Erik used to crack us all up because he looked like Alice Cooper.

The American Cancer Society also sponsored a cosmetic class for people going through chemotherapy and radiation. That was right up Maureen's alley and she learned everything she could about what colors to use to disguise the yellowish skin and the shadows under eyes. She learned over again how to apply false eyelashes for when hers fell out and how to pencil in eyebrows that looked almost real. Every morning Maureen got up and did her face and put on her wig before she woke up the boys.

"Don't worry about them so much. They can take it," I told her one morning.

She looked at me in the mirror. "They don't need to see their mother falling apart," was all she said and she went back to drawing on her eyebrows.

She didn't change her routine for the rest of the house either. She washed and folded the laundry, vacuumed, did the dishes and got after the boys for their homework. She slept on the couch so she could keep an eye on them during the day. Dinner was always ready when I got home, even if it was a frozen pizza. Maureen still picked out our favorites and added a salad to make it seem like a real dinner. Once, I caught her up on a stool with a rag in her hand, but she wasn't moving. I asked her what she was doing.

"These ducks are all dusty, Bill. I've got to clean them."

I took her arm and helped her down. "The ducks can wait, Maureen. They're not going anywhere." I'd like to think I dusted them for her, but I don't remember. I know it bothered her that she couldn't do all the cleaning she used to.

Maureen lost weight too, about fifteen pounds. That might have been the only thing about chemotherapy that made her happy. She never put on a lot of weight, but the last few years she had struggled to lose a few pounds. Now it was coming off all by itself.

Right around this time our church had enough members and enough money to hire a full-time minister. We hired the best minister ever, Reverend Steve Sayer. During one of the first weeks he was there, sometime in early June of 1997, Maureen and I were hanging out on the front porch of the church and she mentioned to Steve that she had just been diagnosed with breast cancer and had been through a treatment already. She said, "Hopefully that's it, it's taken care of." I remember Steve looking at her and sharing her hope. He asked if she needed any-thing, if she would like him to visit, but Maureen was pretty self-contained. She thought she had this thing licked. I remember the whole congregation being hopeful. Our community was so strong, we just knew we could heal her together.

Further biopsies
Medical Record 5/29/97
Biopsy of left axilla—path report negative for malignancy

Medical Record 6/3/97
Office Visits
S/p excision of lymphatic cyst left axilla

At Maureen's next visit, Doctor Schuster found another lump under her arm and did a biopsy right away. He quickly scheduled it to be taken out a few days later. It turned out to be what they call a 'wall cyst', but we were both shaken. When we were getting into the car, Maureen put her head back and blew out like she'd been holding her breath for days.

"If I never hear the word 'lump' again in my whole lifetime, it will be too soon," she said. "How many different kinds of lumps can one person have?"

"I know, Maureen," I told her. "But this one we can forget about. Maybe it's a practice run for forgetting about all the others."

She was well into the chemotherapy by now and the Adriamycin made her throw up. The anti-nausea medicine worked pretty well, but she still had a hard time keeping anything down right after she'd had the chemo. Doctor Mullen started doing regular blood work to find out if the chemo was killing the cells, the good and the bad. Her white counts went down, her red counts went down, her platelets went down. Normal white blood counts for a woman should be 4,500 to 150,000 per micro liter. Normal platelet counts for a woman should be 140,000 to 450,000 per micro liter. Maureen's counts were far below the normal.

Platelets can help restore the blood's clotting ability. They are usually given to people with too few platelets, and if you don't have enough platelets, you can have severe and spontaneous bleeding. Platelets can be stored for only five days. Hemoglobin are oxygen-carrying proteins within the red blood cells.

Women should have 12.5–15 grams per deciliter. Maureen had 9.1.

Maureen struggled on with the Adriamycin and Cytoxan through four regimes, looking forward to radiation afterward. She was determined. She was fighting against what she feared most in her life. But she fought to keep our life normal. We even went camping that summer of 1997. She wouldn't let the cancer keep her from doing anything she normally did. From March to September she went about her life. With all her treatments, worry and pain, Maureen never lost sight of what the boys needed. She never stopped taking them to the places they liked to go. When it was time for the yearly Kneobles and Promised Land camping trip at the beginning of September, Maureen insisted on going just as she was because she didn't want the boys to miss out. She didn't want someone else to take them, because she wasn't ready to give them up. Even though she was in no shape to do it, she went to the amusement park along with everybody else.

Chemotherapy continues
Medical Record 6/10/97
Fourth cycle of Adriamycin & Cytoxan

Medical Record 6/19/97
CT of the abdomen essentially negative
CT of the chest: No evidence of hilar or mediastinal adenopathy.
No pulmonary modules or infiltrates are seen.
No obvious metastatic bony lesion.

Medical Record 7/1/97
CT scans are "clean"
Fifth cycle of Adriamycin & Cytoxan

We rode the rides, but it was not a typical day even though Maureen was pretending it was. The boys went on all the rides, and we worked our way to the back where the roller coaster was. Erik and Ryan wanted to ride the Phoenix roller coaster like we always did while Maureen waited. Not this time. Here came Maureen. She used to be deathly afraid of roller coasters, but now she's facing a bigger fear and fighting like hell. She wanted to be on the roller coaster with Erik and Ryan. They couldn't believe it.

"Mom, what are you doing?"

"I'm riding the Phoenix."

I can't even try to make the faces to show you how excited and happy Erik and Ryan were that their mom was going to go on this roller coaster.

"Oh let me sit with Mom!" They both wanted to sit with their Mom, but it was a two-seater, so Ryan sat with her. Maureen rode in the very first car, the scariest place on a roller coaster. We started off, and Erik sat by me. We were three or four cars behind. I focused on Maureen. I never took my eyes off her. We got up the big hill, and I knew she was going to get blasted. She had never been on a roller coaster and now she's going down this roller coaster that's fast as heck. She started down that hill and she had a smile on her face. Erik and Ryan kept their eyes on Maureen too, knowing this was her first ride. They wanted to see her expression. We zoomed down the hill and off came her wig. Just how fast that roller coaster was going, that's the split second it took for her wig to fly off. And this is no lie; I reached up, three cars back, and caught it. Erik and Ryan could not believe that I caught their mom's wig, I didn't believe it either.

When we got off, Maureen was laughing like I had never seen her laugh. She could barely stand, she was laughing so hard. She was so full of joy, and she wanted to show the boys how strong she was. She put the wig in her purse and got back on that roller coaster and rode it again. The boys were ecstatic, tremendously happy that their mom had ridden the roller coaster with them.

The day was over, and I thought we'd just drive to the campsite at Promise Land. We didn't need anymore stories. I just wanted to get Maureen settled. She was sick and drained. She had ridden an amusement park roller coaster, and she was riding an emotional roller coaster. We pulled out of Kneobles and drove through the little town.

"Bill! Stop!" she yelled all of a sudden. "Look! That's my headstone!"

"What?" I felt like I was in some weird movie.

"Go back! Go back!"

I couldn't believe her, but I did what she asked.

"I just found my headstone."

The boys were there in the car with us and they heard Maureen being honest. She wasn't saying, "I'm going to be all right, I'm going to live." No, she said, "Pull over."

I turned around, and we all got out and walked over to this headstone. It was a beautiful polished granite headstone shaped into a heart. She put her hand on it, looked at me and said, "Bill, I want this headstone for my grave."

The boys didn't say anything. I wanted to cry.

We had just had a pretty good day at Kneobles. But we never really had a good day, we had good moments. And it is the moments that I remember more than the whole day, because the whole day was filled up with crying, throwing up and sickness. So this was going to be a day with some good moments. Maureen found her headstone. We got back in the car and we went to Promised Land campground.

Breast lumps not responding
Medical Record 7/7/97
Emergency visit: c/o severe pain in left arm & left breast
r/o mastitis placed on Duracef

Medical Record 7/14/97
Diflucan was prescribed for a yeast infection after antibiotic therapy

---

The next day, I was sitting outside of our camper, and I heard Maureen say, "Bill come here." It was the same 'Bill come here' that I was used to now. "What's going on?" I asked.

She said "My arm."

Her arm was inflamed and her breast was very hard, like it was when Maureen nursed the boys when they were babies. We hadn't gone far from home or the hospital. We never went far now from anything. We stayed around the community, the church and the hospital. We called Doctor Mullen immediately, and he told us to come in.

Doctor Mullen gave Maureen an antibiotic, Duracef, but it wasn't for a regular infection. The cancer was spreading, and the Adriamycin wasn't working. Maureen was so upset and worried. The doctor told us that sometimes cancer doesn't respond to a particular type of chemotherapy and that we needed to change the chemotherapy to something stronger.

Antibiotics and another biopsy
Medical Record 7/22/97
Persistent swelling left breast,
"she feels that the breast is swollen and the nipple about to crack open ... left breast looks slightly larger and there is definite firmness in the deeper tissues of the breast."
Hold 6th dose of chemo & consult with surgeon
re: possible biopsy

Medical Record 7/24/97
Needle biopsy x 3 left breast
Urinary burning and hematuria-
Bactrum and Diflucan prescribed.

The first antibiotic wasn't strong enough, so they put Maureen on tramoxazole, or Bactrum. Those strong antibiotics gave Maureen a painful yeast infection so she had to take Diflucan also. She was miserable. To make things worse, Maureen's friend Lynn called. They had talked a lot on the phone since Maureen had been diagnosed, and Lynn told me not once did she ever hear Maureen feeling sorry for herself. But Lynn had bad news too.

"I found a lump in my breast, Maureen," she said. "And the doctors told me to go home and not worry about it. What do you think about that?"

"You go back and tell them you want a biopsy," Maureen told her. "Don't take no for an answer."

About ten days later Lynn called back. "I told them to humor me, Maureen. I told them my oldest friend had just been diagnosed with breast cancer."

"Tell me the results, Lynn."

"It's cancer, Maureen. I had three doctors call me back and apologize profusely."

"Do you think they're worried about law suits?" Maureen asked.

"Probably. But the apologies felt good."

Lynn and Maureen followed each other's progress. Lynn ended up having two radical mastectomies. Lynn says, "Because of Maureen, I'm alive today." Maureen was happy to do whatever she could for Lynn.

Maureen talked to the lawyers a few times that summer, but they knew she was fighting for her life. They let her do that while they went about their jobs. I know they started contacting the doctors and sent out requests for records. They told us the records backed up Maureen's story one hundred percent. It was no surprise to us.

New Chemotherapy regime; possible mastectomy
Medical Record 7/25/97
Breast biopsy is positive for cancer.
Chemo switched to Taxol.
May need left mastectomy.

Maureen began taking Taxol. She didn't finish the entire Adriamycin and Cytoxan treatment because the cancer had spread. Taxol is even stronger chemotherapy and it reduces the white and red blood counts even more. It too makes your hair fall out and makes you throw up. Doctor Mullen told Maureen that it might make her joints and muscles achy, even her nerves, and her toes and fingers might get numb. He told her she might get short of breath from the red blood counts going down, causing low blood pressure. All those things happened, but Maureen's hopes rose, because she was getting stronger chemotherapy and the inflammation in her arm went down. The Taxol took the hardness of her breast away. That was good news. If the swelling in her breast could go down, the doctors could do a mastectomy. Until then, her breast cancer was inoperable.

I knew now that Maureen had Stage IV cancer. The disease had taken hold and the doctors were scrambling to get it to slow down. I didn't like keeping secrets, but Maureen had said early on that if it got bad, she didn't want to know. I remembered that doctor that first day saying, "Bill, it's bad." It was so bad the doctor prescribed Vicodin, a narcotic for the pain. It contains pure hydrocordone. I didn't want Maureen in any more pain, so I prayed the Taxol would do its work.

Tumors causing severe pain; chemotherapy continues
Medical Record 7/26/97
Patient called c/o severe breast and arm pain. Vicodin prescribed.

Medical Record 7/29/97
Taxol given

The Taxol had an affect on the bone cancer too. Maureen didn't know that she had bone cancer, because I didn't tell her. She had to fight. Every time Maureen complained of aches in her legs or her stomach, I told her to remember what the doctors had said about the side effects of the chemotherapy. I didn't want to think about what was really going on. I kept praying and so did Maureen. Our whole congregation said prayers every Sunday for her. It was a big shock to them when the first chemotherapy didn't work. Now they all knew that this was going to be a tough fight.

Possible bone cancer
Medical Record 7/30/97
Whole Body Bone Scan:
"some abnormal uptake in the area of the skull, possibly in the basis of metastatic disease."
CT scan of the abdomen and pelvis.

Medical Record 8/1/97
Bone scan shows 2 vague areas in the skull.

Medical Record 8/5/97
Office Visit

They never saw Maureen get angry though. Every Sunday she got up, put on her makeup and fixed her wig. She put on her washed and ironed dress and walked up the aisle with a smile for all her friends. She didn't want anyone to see her giving in or hear her complain. Her conversations about that were with God. She didn't want people to give her pity.

Around this time, Steve Sayer asked her again if she would like him to come and visit. This time Maureen said yes. When he showed up Maureen had on her country music and her makeup. They sat on the couch and talked for over an hour. A couple of times I heard them laughing a little, but Maureen didn't let all her feelings out even with him. I know she told him how disappointed she was about her diagnosis, but she never questioned why it had happened to her. She told him she was afraid for her boys.

Only one time did she really show her anger at how unfair it all was. We were sitting in church, all four of us, and she whispered to me, "I don't feel like God's listening. How many prayers do I have to make? Why is he taking me away from everything I love?"

"Don't say that, Maureen," I said. "Of course he's listening."

"I can't stand it anymore! Why is it me? Why isn't it you or anybody else in this church?" Her face was white and so were her hands gripping the pew in front of her. All of a sudden she got up and walked out of church. I started to follow her and then I knew it was what she needed to do. She walked eight miles home, crying.

Reverend Sayer saw her leave the church and knew she might need someone to talk to. He called and came for a visit that week. She got dressed and made sure her wig was on right before he came, and Garth Brooks was playing on the radio when he came through the door. Maureen didn't want him to see her moping, as she called it. After he and Maureen got through talking, I walked him out to his car and thanked him for his time and care. Then I asked him if there was anything he could tell me to help me take care of her.

"It's a pleasure to spend time with Maureen," he said. "She's worried about her family. That's the main thing on her mind. She's not trying to be noble, but I get the sense that she's really worried about making it through a few more years for the kids, even to see them grow up. She didn't tell me all her feelings, only what's really weighing her down. She's a strong woman who is handling her feelings with incredible dignity, and I don't think she believes it's proper to unload all her worries on anyone.

She's very special, and I'm happy to help, but I think you two know each other better than anyone else." He laughed a little at this point and went on. "You two remind me of Nancy and Ronald Reagan, the way they were so complete in themselves that it seemed like they didn't need anybody else. You have a very tight bond between you, almost like you're complete on your own. I know this illness is drawing you closer, but try to let others in to help. Those who know Maureen need to share in comforting her. Maureen likes to do things properly. Whether it's setting the tables for a fellowship dinner or just taking care to see that the boys' neckties are tied right. She'll want to do this properly too."

It was then that I noticed how carefully Reverend Sayer had dressed for this visit. We shook hands and I went back inside. I teased Maureen that the Reverend looked like an old-fashioned gentleman caller, all spiffed up to see her. She laughed, pleased, then said, "I think it's my fault. We were standing on the church steps one day watching everybody coming in. I saw this man pass by and I said, 'I just hate it whenever I see some guy with an unshaved neck. It doesn't take that much to take care of yourself.' Steve laughed, but I think he took care to have his neck shaved today when he came to the house." It sounds ridiculous, but she had that effect on people. Kind of like keeping the dust off the ducks.

At this point, Maureen started a journal in a little yellow composition book. One of the doctors told her to do that as a way to keep track of what she was going through, but also as a place to put some of her feelings. Maureen was good at looking sturdy on the outside, holding herself together so other people wouldn't have to take care of her. She learned that when she was a kid. But now her feelings were getting the better of her at times. Just like with everything else the doctors told her to do, she got a notebook and started writing in it every day. Most days it wasn't much, but it helped her feel like she was managing at a time when our lives were falling apart. All of Maureen's journal notes are included in a different type with their dates from here on. These passages are all taken directly from her journal.

Chemotherapy continues
Medical Record 8/21/97
Mass in left breast 5-6 cm diameter
Taxol #2 given

Medical Record 8/28/97
Office Visit

Maureen's Journal

8/28/97 Went to lawyer. Also went to GP for finger prick. Feel good. Blood count good.

8/29/97 Going camping. I feel good.

8/30/97 Camping. At peace here. I feel good.

8/31/97 Camping. Resting, reading. Doing good.

9/1/97 Camping. Going home today. Another good day.

9/2/97 School started. Tired, feeling good.

9/3/97 Good day.

9/4/97 Pictures for lawyers today. Feel good.

9/5/97 Good day.

9/6/97 Good day.

9/7/97 Good day.

9/8/97 Good day. A little sore under arm.

She was going through a lot of wigs by that time. The wigs rotted, because the drugs in the chemotherapy ate them. Maureen was on steroids too before and after the Taxol treatments. Those made her bloat and ache in her muscles and joints. She had sore throats from the drugs and she complained of a metal taste in her mouth. Nothing she ate ever tasted good. The chemo drugs were coming out of her pores and she felt nasty all the time after the treatments.

Chemotherapy continues
Medical Record 9/9/97
Taxol #3 given

Maureen's Journal

9/9/97 Chemo. Tired & sore in joints.

9/10/97 Very tired & sore from Chemo & drugs.

9/11/97 Joints sore. Flu-like feeling.

9/12/97 Very, Very, tired. Still sore all over.

9/13/97 Had things to do, but still sore & tired.

9/14/97 Feeling better. I hate chemo.

9/15/97 Sore again under arm. Worry a little. Hope it's nothing.

9/16/97 To the doctor for blood count. See him about sore under arm. Full feeling.

9/17/97 Really scared. Under arm painful. A little depressed. Chemo seems to be working in breast, but underarm feels warm & sore.

9/18/97 Went to see another Oncologist today. Second opinion. She suggests stem cell chemo. Got to fight aggressively. GP called back on pain under arm. CT scan on Wed. He agrees with Oncologist & will look into it for me.

9/19/97 Something is not right. My underarm feels full & numb. I'm always so upset.

All the times that Maureen would be in the hospital or laying on the couch at home, I mean for months, I can't tell you how many times I used to just lay there next to her and try to believe I had some miracle power. You know, something like, "I can do this, I'm going to concentrate and focus on pulling Maureen's cancer out of her body." I'd lay there and pray that her cancer would go from her body to my body. I prayed and prayed and tried drawing this cancer out of her for hours. Just begging God to give it to me. And if God wanted to, I know he could have, without a doubt.

Cat scan and further treatment options
Medical Record 9/18/97
"Still has pain in the left arm ... will get a CT scan at this point ... we need to consider her for stem cell transplant."

Medical Record 9/18/97
Oncologist: Second opinion re: therapy

More opinions
Medical Record 9/19/97
Phone call to physician:
"I suggested that she seek out an opinion with other doctors."

Chapter Four

Stem Cell

We always had hope. Maureen took every visit to the doctor as a step towards her win over cancer. I never heard her say anything that sounded like defeat. Those last reports from the hospital were great, and Maureen was feeling better. Her energy was coming back and she didn't have the pain she had during the summer. Her hair had started to grow back, but the Taxol made it fall out all over again. There was no way that life was anywhere near normal. Some days Maureen's eyes filled up with tears as she watched Erik and Ryan getting ready for school. She hid it from them as best she could. Her hands weren't as busy any more while we watched T.V. or when we went to the lake. All her craft projects had been put aside.

Maureen's Journal

9/20/97 Weekend. Everyone home so I don't think so much of me.

9/21/97 Go to church. I need my faith so much lately.

9/22/97 Just busy at home & always worried about my fate.

9/23/97 Another day. I thank God for each day, but I can't get into things like before the cancer came into my life.

The truth is she was starting to look a lot older, because the chemotherapy was taking its toll. The boys were having a hard time too. I had made my choice to do everything I could to save their mom, but it meant abandoning them. I didn't know what else to do. Nothing was really the same. I took Erik and Ryan for lots of rides so I could try to explain things. They never asked many questions, but sat and listened to how hard their mom was fighting. I don't think they could understand all of it.

On one ride Erik started yelling. "I hate it!" he screamed at me. "We get home from school and the house is dark and cold and dirty. No one's there anymore. At school everybody asks what's going on, and I don't want to answer because I don't want to think about it. I just walk around by myself."

The three of us went quiet. I had nothing to say. I couldn't fix it for them and I couldn't take away what they were feeling. We drove some more and it felt like I was driving through the thickest fog I'd ever been through. Nothing made sense. The teachers at school tried to help. Some of them were wonderful. Ryan's fourth grade teacher, Miss Pile, drove him home once and had dinner with us. She tried to talk to him and help him understand. Another time she brought a whole turkey and came in and ate with the boys while Maureen and I were at the hospital. She called the house from time to time to give Ryan a grownup to talk to. It helped, I know it did, but the truth is, when we were going through it, we were all kind of numb.

I found Maureen in the living room one day crying and tearing up some papers. "What are you doing? What's wrong?" I asked her.

She showed me the torn up scraps. I put the pieces together and saw it was a brochure for a cruise ship. When I looked at her, her eyes were flooded and her mouth was all twisted.

"Aw, Maureen, it's going to be O.K. We'll go on a cruise, just not now. This Taxol seems to be working."

"I know, but I thought by now we could celebrate. I thought we'd be past all this and the breast cancer would just be something we talked about like a hard time we went through. I need some good news, Bill. In all this time, no one has said anything good to me."

She was crying hard, and all I could do was hold her, feel her shaking and let the front of my shirt get soaked.

Results of CAT scan
Medical Record 9/24/97
CT of the chest with contrast:
"no significant change in appearance of the chest compared to the previous CT study of 7/13/97."

Maureen's Journal

9/24/97 2 p.m. CAT scan of chest underarm to see why I'm in pain.

9/25/97 N.C.C.I dinner with K.D ... Saw Mary Beth. Nice dinner. Got on T.V 13. So much cancer around.

9/26/97 O.K. day.

9/27/97 Ryan & Bill go to dentist. Ryan has a filling. I stay home to rest.

9/28/97 Church & family day. I love Bill so much. He's good to me.

9/29/97 Another O.K. day.

9/30/97 Chemo 10 a.m. at GP. Hope this one works.

10/1/97 Tired.

10/2/97 Do Jane's hair, but I'm tired. Nice to talk to her.

10/3/97 Doing a lot of stem cell thinking.

10/4/97 Family is home, so I'm better.

10/5/97 Sunday. Church

10/6/97 See Radiologist to hear his opinion of my breast & stem cell. Real scary stuff. His opinion: "Go for it."

10/7/97 Get blood count & meet surgeon.

Chemotherapy reduces tumor
Medical Record 9/30/97
Office Visit
Mrs. Thiel reports the discomfort in the left breast is significantly better.

Maureen decided that once the boys were back in school, she could spend more time finding other doctors and getting their opinions. It seemed like we talked to everybody. Maureen just kept on going. She wanted all the answers she could find.

Radiology Oncologist recommends next steps
Medical Record 10/7/97
Office Visit: Improvement in left breast.
Radiology Oncologist has suggested a combination of surgery followed by radiation followed by the stem cell transplant.

Maureen's Journal

10/8/97 I'm a wreck. Nervous. I'm in bad shape cancer wise.

10/9/97 See Specialist in Hackensack N.J. 12:45 appt. Left there around 5 p.m. He believes stem cell is about all that is left for me to do. My cancer is bad & there's only a little hope. I go to GP on the way home. Can't stop shaking & crying. Is this the end for me? Oh, God! No one knows how I feel. Doctor gives me nerve pills. They help calm me.

10/10/97 Newton Hospital for CAT scan, bone scan & pulmonary function test. All to get ready for stem cell with specialist.

Maureen had bone cancer with full-blown metastatic breast cancer. This is Stage IV cancer, which means the cancer had spread from her breast to her bones and would probably spread to her lungs, her liver and her brain. The idea now was to keep her alive as long as possible and to ease her symptoms. Her survival chances? Maybe 16%. Maureen was tough, she kept me going. I even believed that she could beat this. And I kept Maureen positive, because she had to stay strong and fight like hell.

But the cancer had spread all through her bones right up her neck to her head; the chemotherapy wasn't working. Maureen decided to get another opinion. We went to Doctor Brooks and Doctor Ames. Doctor Ames said something stronger needed to be done. He said, "This is an aggressive cancer, so we need to fight it aggressively." During this first visit with Doctor Ames Maureen found out that she had 47 positive lymph nodes removed back in April. When we left the appointment Maureen turned to me, her face was like a funeral already happening.

Cancer metastasized to bones
Medical Record 10/10/97
CT scan of the Abdomen and Pelvis:
"Extensive metastatic disease now present in the skeleton, otherwise no change from the study of 7/30/97.
Whole Body Bone Scan: "the patient now has disseminated metastatic disease involving much of the spine, pelvis, both hip regions, both rib cages as well as the skull and neck.

"Why didn't you tell me?" where her first words. No hug.

I knew right away. I stood there making myself look at her. I had never told her one lie in the whole time we'd been together and now she caught me in the biggest lie you could tell a person. "I wanted to give you a chance."

"A chance? How am I supposed to have a chance, if I don't even know what I'm dealing with?"

"I didn't want them telling you some numbers that meant you'd give up. I thought if I could hold off the numbers, the reports, it would give you room to try to live."

We weren't shouting, but our voices had points and the heaviness of big stones. We just stood squeezed on either side of the hard space between us.

Maureen moved first. She stepped toward me slowly, trying to shrink the blank nothing of our fear and she put herself into my arms. "I can never give up. Not on you and me."

We stood cradling each other, heads together. "Tell me," I said. "Tell me what you want."

"Stem cell therapy," Maureen said, and those words began the next months of our life. After that day, I wasn't going to let her go anywhere without me. We went to the specialist to hear what this new treatment was all about. It meant even more aggressive chemotherapy and then a transplant of Maureen's stem cells. All of Maureen's doctors agreed that if she was a good candidate, then stem cell was something she should try. We went to Hackensack, New Jersey, and met the doctors there.

The stem cell therapy specialists explained the whole set of procedures to us. Maureen came out of there so upset and scared. It was all they had left for her. The doctors told us we had no more choices, and only if Maureen was a candidate. What's a candidate? A good candidate has good health insurance to cover the cost. Not all insurance companies will cover a stem cell transplant. There's a lot of talk right now in the news about stem cell research and many people don't understand what stem cell is or what the pros and cons might be. Anyone in Maureen's shoes wouldn't see the negative side of the argument, because it might be the only thing to save her life. I wanted her to have a chance. Insurance companies shouldn't make the choice, because the treatment does work.

Maureen's Journal

10/11/97 Go food shopping with the family. I'm nesting & afraid of missing them.

10/12/97 Go to church. Bill breaks down & asks people to pray for me. Ray & Teresa are there & we go to breakfast with them.

10/13/97 11:00 a.m. appt. to meet surgeon to see what he says about breast removal & to get Quinton catheter in my chest. Breast can not be removed. Tumor too large. He can do the catheter whenever I need it. Nice guy. Where is God? I pray & beg & hope all the time for good news. Bill tells me the bone scan showed specks in my bones. So the cancer is spreading. But I still have to fight this devil.

10/14/97 Go to dentist. Pulls a $600 root canal molar with a cap. Very painful.

Before Maureen could go through stem cell therapy, she had to have a tooth pulled. Her dentist removed the tooth rather than do a full root canal he had planned. There wasn't enough time for the root canal, and Maureen couldn't risk an infection. It seemed like little bits of Maureen were coming undone every day. When she came out of the dentist, she wouldn't look at me. Then she almost shouted, "It's only a tooth, Bill! I'm not going to sit here and cry over it." I put the car in gear and drove her home.

Maureen's Journal

10/15/97 Want to stay in bed all day. Reverend Sayer calls & comes over in afternoon. So I get up & we have a nice talk. We pray.

10/16/97 Got appt. with gynecologist in Milford at 10:50 a.m. All this is prep for stem cell. Came right home. Lawyers come to film a deposition.

The lawyers were still in touch. They knew Maureen was fighting hard. Marcia talked with her the most. But the lawyers respected what Maureen had to do. Malcolm told me, "Bill, you're fight is for her life. You fight that fight. We'll fight the legal fight.' And that's what the lawyers focused on. But they didn't know how bad it was until I called them in September and said, "Things are not going great." Malcolm, Marcia and Mike decided to meet with Maureen at the house. I think they were surprised when they saw her. It was the first time they saw her beaten down. She was sad.

They interviewed her and made a legal deposition on videotape right in our living room. Maureen answered all their questions and stayed focused. Marcia asked her how she felt about everything she was going through and how she felt about leaving her kids. It was only then that she cried and it wasn't for herself; it was for Erik and Ryan. At the end, she looked right into the camera and said, "I just hope every woman insists and checks. If I live through this, I will become an advocate so everybody knows how to do breast exams. Everybody should insist, don't let doctors tell you 'wait, don't worry.' You've got to get a biopsy. You've got to know right away. I told Bill, that's what I'm going to do with my life if I make it. I've learned that 40,000 women die each year of breast cancer, so I want to tell this story on Oprah to try to help those women."

Maureen's Journal

10/17/97 Bill is out of work now. He just can't cope any more. Seems he <u>has</u> to be with me. I feel for Bill. He's a wonderful person to me. At 11:00 we go back to N.J. to the dentist for a filling. 1 p.m. I have an appt at J.T.L. School with Erik's teachers to inform them of what's going on at home. They are all caring & will help. I rush to pick up some food, then from J.T.L. we stop to get Ryan & we're off to Milford for an E.T. booster shot. We eat out, then home & I am so tired. So many doctors & so many miles.

10/18/97 Sat. I rest, but off to flee market to do some Christmas shopping for boys, in case I can't do it later.

10/19/97 Sunday. Church is my salvation. The people are real & make me feel loved & cared for. I was going to walk with K.D in the cancer walk at Liberty Park, but it may rain & it is so cold, so I stayed home. I raised $146. She raised close to $700 & she did the 5-mile walk.
10/20/97 Went to Morristown Hospital for pre-testing: blood & E.K.G. Bill took me out to lunch.

The type of stem cell they wanted Maureen to have is called Adult Stem Cell Transplant, or Autologous Transplant, meaning that Maureen would donate her own bone marrow before she had the high-dose chemotherapy. In the body, bone marrow holds the stem cells, which are multi-purpose cells that can become other types of specialized cells, like red and white blood cells and platelets.

The doctors explained it to us like this: The brain knows how many cells it needs every day throughout the whole body. It sends a chemical message to the stem cells in the bone marrow. The stem cells are like tadpoles. They're stupid cells, not anything useful yet. But when they get the message from the brain, it tells them what kind of cells they should be. So the brain might send a message saying it needs 110,015 red blood cells, 22,908 white blood cells and 43,211 platelet cells. The stem cells sort themselves out and develop into the kind of cells the brain has ordered. Having a strong, cancer-free supply of stem cells was critical after all the cancer cells had been killed by the chemotherapy. Those clean stem cells were going to go in and rebuild Maureen.

The sequence of the treatments during the stem cell therapy was complicated. First we would go to Morristown Hospital in New Jersey to have a Double Quinton catheter installed in Maureen's chest. Next we would go to Newton Memorial in New Jersey, but closer to home, for a bone aspiration to see if Maureen's stem cells were clear of cancer. Then the real stem cell therapy could begin.

The first phase would be at Newton Memorial Hospital. Maureen would receive high-dose chemotherapy and then wait for her platelet, white and red blood counts to come back up. Then the second phase could begin. She would go to Hackensack, New Jersey, where they would remove the clear stem cells using a phoresus machine. The second phase involved more, high-dose chemotherapy at Hackensack. Once that chemotherapy was done, they would reintroduce healthy stem cells and wait for them to graft. The final step was to begin doses of the drug Neumega or Neupogen to help increase Maureen's blood platelet and white blood counts. Neumega was still in clinical trials at that time.

The first thing her regular doctor had to do was check Maureen to see if her body was a good candidate for stem cell replacement therapy. He did a bone scan, a CAT scan, a lung scan to check her pulmonary functions, and an EKG to see if her heart could make it through. She had to lie still for two hours while they did an MRI to check everything else. She went to the gynecologist for a pap smear to make sure there were no infections. He also checked her mouth for sores.

She was ready. Everything was set to begin. The sky was a milky blue, and I was waiting for her outside the house. I knew she was making her rounds, checking all the faucets, the stove, the kids' room windows and the locks on the door. I knew today she'd check them more than twice. Maureen opened the front door and saw me in the yard holding the video camera. She didn't say anything, just walked straight toward me and stopped.

"One more stone," she said. She tapped her foot on a grassy spot between two flat steppingstones. "One more, right here." She pointed down at her tapping toe and laughed.

I held the video camera so her face filled the lens, her wide smile with lipstick, her thick eyelashes and the crinkles at the corners of her eyes.

"Look down," she said, giving her throaty laugh again.

I pointed the camera down and she tapped her toe for the movie. When I brought the camera up again, her eyebrow was arched and the smile had softened. "Don't forget." She turned and walked back along the stones and up the steps to the car. She paused before she got in and looked back at the blue clapboards, the owl wind chime beside the door, the apple tree leaves turning to rust.

I zoomed in to catch her close up. Her eyes were still clear, but her mouth was set. She watched a chipmunk skitter around the corner in the dry leaves, took a long, slow breath, then looked right into the lens and lowered herself into the car.

I pressed 'stop' and put the lens cap on, but not before stating clearly for the microphone: "October 22, 1997. Today we begin high-dose chemotherapy for stem cell treatments."

We pulled away and neither of us spoke. We took the familiar roads that ordinarily would have taken us to the community center, to church or to my job at the outdoor equipment distributor. We rounded the curves of small roads that drop away suddenly to stony-bedded creeks or rise abruptly to new growth where old farm fields lay between dry-stacked stone walls. We cut through the Delaware Water Gap and crossed at Dingmans Bridge to the Jersey side of the river. On Route 206 we passed the New Jersey State Fair Grounds, Culver Lake and Osterman's Hardware Store. We were silent. I counted the traffic lights and Maureen lifted her eyes to the pale outline of Kittatinny Mountain with Jenny Jump Mountain behind, deep russet and burnt orange as the sun began to spray our shoulders with light.

Preparation for stem cell therapy
Medical Record 10/20/97
Morristown Memorial Hospital
Outpatient lab work drawn

Before the stem cell team could begin, they added a double Quinton catheter with four valves into Maureen's chest. This was a larger set of tubes that could handle all the drugs they were going to put into Maureen. They also used this type of catheter because it makes it possible to increase the number of stem cells circulating in the blood after the chemotherapy. The porta-cath in her chest that had two valves was still there.

The specialist in charge of the stem cell chemotherapy told us what kind of drugs Maureen was going to get. She would still get the Cytoxan and the Taxol that she had been taking before, but now she was going to have them together. After that she was going to get Platinol. At Newton Memorial Hospital Maureen was going to be the pioneer patient for stem cell chemotherapy, so all the medical staff had to learn in a hurry. They asked as many questions as we did. I heard one nurse say when she looked at Maureen's chart, "Oh my God, what is this?" Maureen was Doctor Mullen's first stem cell patient. He told me, "Bill you're just going to have to educate yourself." In the library, I had my own cubicle, and the librarians helped. I read constantly and got eyestrain. Maureen had 64 different drugs during stem cell. I had a chart to keep track.

Maureen's Journal

10/21/97 Well, it's all starting. Today is the day. Morristown at 11:15. Surgery at 12:45 for Quinton Catheter. Left recovery at about 3 to come to Newton. I'm admitted. GP does bone marrow aspiration. I'm so tired from driving, blood work & surgery, but I can't sleep. Nerves. K.D., my sister, is with the boys. I must mention K.D. is helping a lot. She'll be there for the boys. I'm trying to enroll them in Cranford N.J. schools. They'd live with Mom & K.D. This way it's not so much running & the boys going from house to house. When you're scared & depressed because you're facing possible death it's nice to know you're loved & cared for & that you'd be missed.

10/22/97 I have not slept much. Chemo starts at 8 a.m. today.

Catheter Surgery
Medical Record 10/21/97
Morristown Memorial Hospital
Placement of Double Lumen
Right Subclavian Pheresis Catheter
(QuintonCatheter)

High Dose Chemotherapy
Medical Record 10/22/97
Newton Memorial Hospital
Bone Marrow Aspiration:
no metastatic tumor cells are noted.
High dose chemotherapy:
Cytoxan 3750 mg x 2 days,
Cisplatin 60 mg x 2 days,
Atoposide 750 mg x 3 days.

They did the bone marrow aspiration in an operating room, and Maureen was wide awake for that. They gave her an epidural to block the pain from her back, but I don't think there was anything they could have given her that would have stopped her from feeling what they were doing. The doctors took out the stem cells by sticking large needles, which looked like steel rods, into the sacroiliac region of her back. That's the very lowest part of the backbone. They kept turning and turning that rod and I could almost hear the grinding. Maureen screamed through the whole procedure. With the needles they took out samples of the stem cells from the bone marrow. The lab took the sample and tested it to see if there was any evidence of cancer. The news that came back was good. No evidence of cancer in the stem cells.

While the high-dose chemotherapy kills the cancer cells, it kills just about everything else along with it. Before Maureen could begin stem cell therapy she had to sign papers. If she died on the table, the hospital was not at fault, because they are lethal doses of chemicals. The drugs are cytotogenic, tertogenic and carcinogenic. They are highly toxic. Maureen was told that, and she signed all the papers.

Maureen's Journal

10/23/97 Chemo is intense. Can hardly breathe nor sleep. I feel sick & scared. Why is this happening?

10/24/97 Too sick to think. I feel dead.

10/25/97 Morning horrible. They pump that stuff in so fast, I feel my heart giving up. I go home today, but I'm scared. Can't sleep or breathe.

Maureen was blasted with chemo. I'll never forget the table with all the drugs on it. I sat waiting for the chemotherapy to begin at Newton Hospital and an orderly pushed a big table full of drugs past me. Our nurse was waiting with me and she saw the table too. It was a whole table of chemotherapy drugs. This hospital was not new to chemotherapy, they were used to giving out drugs, and they had lots of experience with cancer patients.

The nurse beside me said, "That's the most chemotherapy I've ever seen. How many people are getting treatments today?"

She thought the doses were for everyone on that hospital floor. It was all for Maureen. That nurse had been there many years, and she couldn't believe it. She had never seen anything like it before. And the head nurse had never seen it either. When they looked the order over, they thought it was a mistake. But it wasn't. The drugs they gave Maureen made a toxic soup.

A normal dose of Cytoxan might be 300 or even 500 mg for Maureen's body weight. They gave her 3,750 mg. Twice. They also gave her two other cancer drugs after that. Platinol or Cisplatin suppresses the production of platelets in the body. It's hard on the kidneys and has all kinds of side effects. It takes about 40 days to recover, but before recovery, the affect on the renal system is severe. It caused Maureen's face to swell, her lungs to constrict and she couldn't taste anything for weeks after. Her legs cramped up too. Thankfully she never lost her hearing or had any blurred vision. They told us those could be side effects too.

Atoposide or Etoposide interferes with cancer cells, but it also decreases the body's ability to fight infections. For a short time after it's been injected it reduces how many blood cells the bone marrow makes. That drug was a whopper too. Maureen's heart started racing and her breath got short. There was a whole list of other possible side effects like loss of consciousness, bleeding, numbness in fingers and toes, difficulty walking. I learned that some side effects might not happen until months or even years after they had given her the medicine.

The platelets are killed off as well as healthy cells. The platelets are usually at their lowest 18 to 23 days after you get the drugs and don't get back to healthy numbers until maybe 39 days. For some people it takes as long as 62 days to get back to normal. The doctors told us about the side effects. Of course nausea and vomiting was at the top of the list along with hair loss. This was phase one of Maureen's chemotherapy. Those nurses called Hackensack Medical Center and contacted the nurses over there to make sure this was all correct. Newton Memorial had to learn fast. The staff at Hackensack Medical coached them on how to proceed.

Maureen had five doses of this chemo and each one took twelve hours. Those first few days, from surgery for the double Quinton, to getting more blood tests done, to another hospital for more tests, and back to the original hospital for the bone marrow aspiration, was like a whole year's worth of episodes on the television show *ER*. As soon as they took out the bone marrow, we started the chemo part of the stem cell therapy. Maureen was just crushed by it. It was wicked.

I never left Maureen's side. I was quarantined throughout the whole thing right along with her. In the recovery room, she came to a little. She looked like hell. I wasn't even going to ask her how she felt. But she told me.

"It was like a dump truck just dumped all the garbage into the landfill of my chest."

Maureen started throwing up and she never stopped. She thought she was going to die and so did I. The nurse that usually took care of many patients on a twelve-hour shift, now just took care of Maureen. She never left the room. If she did, I was there. I wasn't leaving, and I hardly closed my eyes all during that time. I went days without sleeping. Every patient had to have a caregiver while they stayed in the outpatient wing of the hospital. I was Maureen's caregiver. I took Maureen's temperature several times a day and wrote it down in a notebook. I got Maureen her bed pan and her throw up bucket. I changed her nightgown and her underpants. I washed her the best I could and I listened to moans that told me she was in pain. I tried not to miss anything Maureen's body was trying to tell me.

Then I took her home. She had been through hell in the hospital, and neither of us could wait to get out of there, but the idea of being at home was terrifying. Maureen had no immune system. She couldn't be around fresh fruit or flowers; she couldn't be near anybody without a mask over her nose and mouth, and she had to wash her hands before and after she did anything. Maureen threw up all the time and the smell was unbelievable. She was so sick. She had another phase of the stem cell therapy to go through, but not until her blood counts came up. I wasn't sure if she was going to make it through the second phase. But she wanted to live for Erik and Ryan.

She was so weak when she came back from the hospital after the first phase, but after a while she actually felt better, she rebounded, and her counts came back up. She was tough. She made it through the first phase at Newton Memorial Hospital and then got ready to face the final phase of chemotherapy at Hackensack. In the second phase, they would remove the stem cells, freeze them, give Maureen more chemotherapy, then put the stem cells back into her body and hope that they graft. Once the re-introduced stem cells graft, the blood counts come back up and the cancer should be gone. That was the plan.

Maureen's Journal

10/26/97 Sunday. Bill & Erik go to church. I'm home with K.D. & Ryan. I eat a cup of Jello. Oh God! I'm in labor-like state for 2 hours. Can't breathe. Feel so sick. Finally throw up & I feel a bit better. Nurse comes to teach shots. Patty Flotz comes to learn how. This whole thing is awful, but it's all I've got.

Building Platelets
Medical Record 10/25/97
Discharged with instructions to start Epogin 480 mg twice a day.

Medical Record 10/26/97
Instructed husband and friend on proper subcutaneous injection technique for Neupogen. Instructed husband on care and flushing of catheter lines.

When we left the Newton Memorial, the doctors prescribed Neupogen shots to keep Maureen's white blood cells up. She had to give them to herself, but she couldn't, because she hated needles. She was tough, but she hated needles, mice, and roller coasters.

Maureen was afraid to let me do it, because she was afraid I would hurt her, so she asked Patty Flotz if she would mind doing it. Patty met one of the hospital nurses at our house and learned about the Neupogen and how to administer the shots. She gave Maureen the first injection. Patty wasn't a nurse, but she wanted to learn and later took phlebotomy courses to become a nurse's assistant. But soon we were advised not to have Patty give the shots because Maureen's immune system was so weak, and Patty had kids and could contaminate Maureen. Patty showed me how, and I gave Maureen most of the rest. As long as she needed injections or porta-caths cleaned or double Quintons cleaned, I did it. Being Maureen's caretaker was my job.

I learned how to clean the catheters and change Maureen's dressings. I made sure nothing got wet or dirty, by keeping the hole in her chest covered with sterile gauze or a special dressing called a vascular access dressing. At one point, I was changing the plugs on the catheter, which are the little valves that allow the medication to go in and not spill out. I was concentrating on doing it right without hurting Maureen, when I realized she was watching me and smiling.

"What are you smiling about?" I asked her.

"You look like you know what you're doing. Like you're having fun tinkering around with my machinery."

"I'm just trying to take care of you right."

"I know. I don't want anyone else playing with my valves."

We both busted up laughing. I couldn't believe her, lying there with tubes coming out of her chest, her hair all gone and her face tired as an old woman's, and still she's giving me that light in her eyes. If her body could have taken it, I would have curled up next to her and held her the way I always had.

The next phase of treatment involved removing stem cells, and for that Maureen needed to go to Hackensack, New Jersey. She was also still getting transfusions all the time, so we wore a path back and forth to both Newton Memorial and Hackensack. After the stem cells were removed, another round of high-dose chemotherapy would begin and we would be quarantined at Hackensack hospital for two months or three months. Once she began the treatment, she couldn't leave. During this phase, the boys changed schools and stayed with Maureen's mother and her sister Kathryn. It felt horrible splitting up the family, but it was all we could think of to do. At least they came home on weekends before Maureen went into quarantine, and we tried to make up for the days in between. One weekend, they told Maureen they were roller-blading in skate parks. She hated that. Erik was the skate boarder and Ryan was the roller blader. I think it kept them from going crazy and they got pretty good at it. But they knew Maureen wasn't happy about it. It was one more thing that she couldn't control. She couldn't tell them to stop, because she wasn't there to make her words stick.

The boys always looked so scared when they visited, and I know neither one of them liked being away from home. Erik told me once it felt like our family had been stolen. They had each other though. Just like any kids, they made the best of what was happening. They stayed in the attic at Maureen's mother's and one night they started a pillow fight. I guess they made a mess, with their mattresses all over. Their Aunt Katheryn came up to see what was going on and she slipped in all the feathers. She knew the boys needed to blow off some steam. Everybody was having a tough time, but we made those changes so the boys would be closer to Maureen when she went into Hackensack.

Maureen's Journal

10/27/97 My kids are gone. Last night K.D. took them to New Jersey to start school there today. I'm scared for them, because I really don't know what this is really doing to them. I love them. I go to GP today. The sun hurts my eyes. My insides feel poisonous. At the doctor's Nurse Kathy cleans all the tubes in me & checks blood. I'm sick again. Can't keep food down & all the smells of medicine & people upset me.

10/28/97 Back to GP to check blood. Still getting sick.

10/29/97 Having a "Pray" for me at church today. Got to go to GP every day to check blood counts. Not sick today.

Through everything, the people from our church never let us down. Most people go for an hour or so and go home. At this church no one wanted to go home, because it was full of great families and people with loving hearts. This community took care of not just Maureen, but the boys and me too. They brought bags and bags of food, and whole dinners so the boys and I wouldn't have to cook. The community and her best friends were always thinking of what they could do to help us.

Maureen still needed a lot of transfusions, so the hospital asked me to donate blood. Her platelet count wasn't rising fast enough. She slept nearly all day, partly because she was so weak, but also because when she was awake, her mind went over and over everything. She was trying to face what was happening, but it was too much. When she was sleeping, I didn't see the worry and fear that was eating her up.

Maureen's Journal

10/30/97 GP sends us to hospital. My blood counts are dropping fast.

10/31/97 GP & back to hospital. Sit & wait is all I do. Can't see people. Can't go into stores or crowds. Just sit in car & watch life pass by me. It's like a prison sentence. Got to get a transfusion, so I go into hospital at about 3:30 p.m.. I'm here all night. I get home 1:30 a.m.. I'm so tired & weary.

Platelet transfusion
Medical Record 10/30/97
Platelet transfusion for thrombocytopenia

11/1/97 Saturday. I get to stay home. I get tired of going. I don't talk much. Nothing to say. Can't look back & I have no future. I miss my boys.

11/2/97 Bill goes to church. House is so quiet. I feel better than one week ago, but I feel sorry for me. I'm a victim right now. No hair, no lashes, no brows, no energy, no social life, no kids. It's got to work.

11/3/97 Trish brings over T.W. of chicken soup. Back to GP. Kathy, the nurse, changes dressing & takes more blood. Go back to hospital & wait alone in car for hours. Don't have to stay, so go home. Nose bleeds a lot. Stomach is tender & where Bill gives me shots is bruising. Told Dr. it's O.K.

11/4/97 Went back to GP. Nurse Kathy took blood & I went back to hospital to wait. Got to come home. Spoke to my boys again tonight. Thank the Lord they're doing good with the living arrangements & school. But I still miss them so much. After talking to them, my legs felt tender so Bill rubbed them & I was walking around the house, but my right leg was in a lot of pain & couldn't put much pressure on it. Bill got a heating pad & I took a pain pill.

11/5/97 Went to GP. Told Nurse Kathy about my legs & spots on my foot. (Reteacia) on foot due to low blood levels. Put me in a wheel chair & sent to hospital for x-rays of the bones. Had to stay for another transfusion.

Steve Sayer visited Maureen many times during these weeks, and it wasn't because Maureen was questioning her faith. She talked to him about helping us so we could go on. I think the hard part for Reverend Sayer and the congregation was that Maureen was the first person to become so sick after all the fellowship work we had done. Of course people become ill in a church community, but Maureen was the first one to have such a serious illness. Everyone saw the tragedy of it: a young woman with two young kids. As in any family, when an elderly relative passes away, that's very sad, but not unexpected, but when it's your sister facing death, that's almost impossible to believe. Folks were shaken. All those people prayed for her for months.

When her platelets were very low, the doctors told Maureen she had thrombocytopenia, which is the body trying to operate without anywhere near enough platelets. Thrombocytopenia happens when the platelet count falls below 50,000. Maureen's platelet counts and her white blood counts kept dropping. She needed transfusions all the time, but the problem with platelets is that after they are donated, they can only be stored for five days.

Platelet transfusion
Medical Record 11/5/997
Admission for transfusion of platelets due to severe thrombocytopenia from chemo

---

We had learned during the first phase at Newton Memorial that Maureen couldn't be around other patients because her immune system was so weak. Whenever we arrived or left even for a transfusion, the nurses cleared the hallways and made sure the elevators were empty. Maureen didn't have anything in her that could fight off germs and infections. The chemotherapy had killed it all.

Maureen's Journal

11/6/97 Back to GP to check blood. Was told Friday to go to Hackensack.

A healthy woman should have a white blood count (WBC) of about 4,500 to 10,500 per microliter. Her platelet count should be 140,000 to 450,000 per micro liter. Maureen's count was 65,000. She would have to be on the machine for three hours to get a small bag of platelets. For some reason, the doctors thought I had great platelets, but after a while they wouldn't let me donate because I got weak and sick. So the church and the neighborhood came to bat. Droves of people came to donate. Some couldn't donate, but they tried. The church folks would say a prayer with me. All of them came to Hackensack, two hours away, to donate platelets, white blood cells, red blood or whole blood, and they were happy to do it for Maureen.

Blood count
Medical Record 11/6/97
Blood count: WBC is 10.0
Platelet count is 65K

Maureen's Journal

11/7/97 Went to Hackensack to remove stem cells. Took 2 ½ hours on machine. What a feeling. Lips went numb. Then hands & feet felt the vibrations of the machine. Got very cold & a little scared. Called the boys when we got home. Ryan hurt his arm.

Removing the stem cells wasn't as bad as the bone aspiration. But it was sickening to watch the life almost literally being drained out of Maureen. She had more than two quarts of fluid removed while she sat in a big reclining chair. The machine behind her looked like a juke box with lights and mechanical arms. But there wasn't any music, just a dull hum that would have put anyone to sleep if it hadn't been sucking the life out of them. Maureen was pale and her eyes were huge the whole time. I kept expecting her to pass out. In a way I kept wishing she would, so she wouldn't be scared any more. She kept herself going by saying little prayers and then pretending she was singing songs to Erik and Ryan.

Maureen's Journal

11/8/97 Saturday went to see boys at my Mom's. Bill took Ryan to hospital. He broke his arm. I felt good except got an itchy rash. Called GP. He said to stop a certain medication & take Benedryl.

Lab results from Cell Specimen
Medical Record 11/7/97
Fresh Peripheral blood stem Cell Specimen submitted to
Laboratories.
Conclusion: "no cells with breast carcinoma present."

11/9/97 Stayed at Mom's with boys. I was very tired & slept most of the day. Bill took them bowling. I really miss being normal. When I am done with all this I am going to be an advocate for breast cancer. O. P. Winfrey P.O. Box 909, 715 Chicago IL 60690. 312 591 9595.

11/10/97 Bill took Ryan to orthopedic doctor for a cast in morning. Erik went off to school. Got all that done & I had to go to Hackensack at 2. On the machine for the stem cells again. Thank goodness they got a lot on this Friday & this would be the last for me. I hate the machine. I hate the feeling you get.

We had proof that all those prayers had been answered. We had a report from the doctors that the removed stem cells were free of cancer. Those words "no cells with breast carcinoma present," were the best words Maureen and I had heard since last April. We were back on track. Maureen was still weak and sick, and now she knew her body was fighting for life.

No cancer present
Medical Record 11/10/97
Fresh Peripheral Blood Stem Cell specimen submitted to
Laboratories
Conclusion: "no cells with breast carcinoma present."

Maureen's Journal

11/11/97 Stayed home today. All I do is sleep. Bill went to work. I got a little sentimental. I miss the kids so much. I'm scared because next week I go to Hackensack for chemo. So much can go wrong. I pray.

11/12/97 Went to GP. Kathy tested blood, then went to hospital to wait, but didn't need transfusion. I'm really speechless these days.

11/13/97 Went to Cranford N.J. this morning to get kids. Now it's better. I love my boys Erik & Ryan. I'm still crying inside. I feel like I'm living my last weekend. I'm kissing the boys like it's my last. I'm so scared of losing them. I want to see them become men.

11/14/97 Snow arrived today. We all stayed in. Icy snow. But I enjoyed my boys. Cut their hair. Lots of hugs. Watch T.V., movies. Sat close. Erik sleeps on the living room floor next to me on the sofa. I pray to God he lets me continue to live my life with my family.

11/15/97 Another good day. I got my boys. I never loved them so much as I do now. I'm so scared for my life. I feel as if this is the last weekend I get to spend with my family. This afternoon we went to the mall. Went out to eat. Gosh the boys ate so many crab legs. Then we went to other stores. Got the boys nice boots & other things, socks, etc. I also did some Christmas shopping. Came home & got things together for the boys. Erik & Ryan slept with me tonight. When I woke I was shaking. This is my last day with them. I lay down between them & we held hands.

11/16/97 Sunday. Erik & Ryan & I woke holding hands. They are so much to me. My fight for life is in their honor. I want to come back for them. I need them. I got their stuff ready to go back to N.J. with Aunt Kathy. The kids saw their friends Johnny & Eddie for a while, then they came home to me. E.T. & I went out. I bought them some baseball & basketball cards. We ate lunch then Erik, Ryan & I read *The Little Engine that Could* & *Teddy Beddy.* We prayed together, hugged, kissed, & I told them I love them & to be good for me. Then they left at 6:30 p.m.. I pray I see them become men. Oh, God, please!

Maureen slept on the couch all the time now. Lots of mornings I found Erik asleep on the floor next to her. He was trying to take care of her and protect her. The night before the boys headed to New Jersey to stay with their Aunt Katheryn, Maureen fell asleep on the floor between Erik and Ryan. She told me after they drove away that she woke up in the middle of the night shaking and couldn't control her nerves. Finally she fell asleep for a few hours and when she woke up again they were all holding hands, sleeping on the floor.

Reverend Sayer still came by for visits, although sometimes Maureen would be too tired. He knew it was time to leave when he saw her shoulders droop a little or she got quiet. One of the last times he came to the house, I heard Maureen and him laughing a little toward the end of their conversation. When I asked her about it later, Maureen said, "Oh, he asked me if I was having trouble being positive. I said, 'Well, I don't know if we're being positive or thick headed, but we're putting on a sun porch. Bill's putting up sheetrock while I'm putting up a fight.' He liked that a lot. Then he looked at me and said, 'If anybody could make it through this, you can.'" At that point Maureen started to cry. "Bill, what's going to happen to the boys? How are they going to hold together? I need to know they're going to be all right."

Even the Reverend Sayer couldn't take away that fear. But he did what he could along with every one else. Meals still showed up at our house, meals that Maureen mostly could never eat. But it wasn't the food that was important, it was all those good people showing us they cared, and it helped. Sometimes it seemed like no amount of prayers was going to work.

On the eve of the second high-dose chemotherapy and quarantine in Hackensack, the church held a 24-hour prayer vigil. I believe prayer has enormous healing power. What could be better than talking to Jesus? I don't know. Everyone signed up. Every hour for twenty-four straight hours someone sat in the church, sometimes two and three people were there because so many people wanted to pray for Maureen.

Maureen's Journal

11/17/97 Slept with Bill last night. We clean up the house. This morning is sunny & bright. I'm waiting for the hospital to call. Today is the day. I cry a lot in fear. But I keep saying I think I can, I think I can & I'm entering the ring for the biggest fight of my life. I love you, Erik. I love you, Ryan. Oh, Bill, thank you for being a wonderful husband. I love you.
XXXXXXXXXXXXXXXXXXXXXXXXXXXXXXXXXXX.
Went to Hackensack. Left home around 4 p.m.. When we got there went to room & it all began. Within an hour a catheter was put in my neck. It hurt. 3 tubes of chemo went into that. 2 more in my chest & a urine catheter was put in. The chemo began. It didn't stop until 10:30 p.m.

Off we went again for the second phase and back into quarantine. Maureen was scared to death. The second phase was the stem cell infusion, and the whole procedure was laid in front of us. This time they gave me the papers to sign in case she died. I signed pretty much everything now. They wouldn't have been able to understand Maureen's signature anyway, because she couldn't stop shaking with fear. The first phase of the chemotherapy had almost killed her and this second phase was supposed to be much worse.

The morning Maureen began the high-dose chemotherapy, the nurses put Maureen on a gurney and started to wheel her to the surgery room. Out in the hall other nurses were bringing a woman from the next room back from the same stem cell procedure. I heard them all talking and trying to hurry, and I figured out pretty quickly that the woman was dead because her heart had given out during the chemotherapy. I moved as fast as I could around the table and got between the other woman and Maureen so she wouldn't see.

Maureen went through the treatment with about eleven other people. Along with the double Quinton catheter, the doctors put in more access lines to her body. Then they added another catheter to her neck to make a total of seven pathways to pour in the drugs

Maureen was given high doses of Cyclophosphamide, or Cytoxan, again. She also got Carboplatin, which is a platinum drug that interferes with cancer cells. It also interferes with normal body cells and causes tiredness, nausea, risk of infection, numbness in hands and feet, hair loss, rashes, dizziness, sores in the mouth, diarrhea, confusion, ringing in the ears, bruising and bleeding, and blurry vision. Then there was Thiotepa. This drug is classified as "Dangerous Goods" under the

Transportation of Dangerous Goods Act. When I looked it up, I discovered that it is mutagenic and carcinogenic, not recommended to be mixed with other drugs, and is incompatible with Cisplatin. This drug produces breaks in the DNA molecules and then cross-links some of the twin strands. The side effects, besides the usual chemotherapy effects, are life threatening because of anaphylaxis and seizures. Anaphylaxis is an allergic reaction that can start with the heart beating faster, feeling uneasy, blood pressure falling, hives, swelling and severe difficulty breathing.

Along with the chemotherapy drugs, there was a host of others. Maureen took Mannitol, which reduces pressure in the brain and is usually used to treat patients with kidney failure. She also took large doses of Decadron, a glucorticoid that acts as an anti-inflammatory. Included was Heparin, which inhibits blood clotting, as well as Lasix, which helps with edema or swelling related to congestive heart failure. Compazine was always around to help with the nausea along with Kytril. And they gave Maureen Ativan to help her anxiety. On top of that were lots of topical ointments for rashes, mouth rinses and vitamins. Each day was a pharmacist's delight and a challenge for the nurses to keep track.

Maureen stayed again in the hospital wing that resembled a hotel, but had all the things a patient needed. We were now under the strictest quarantine at Hackensack, and the days dragged by waiting for Maureen's strength to come back. That November, Erik a band concert, and Maureen was determined not to miss it. She begged the doctors to let her go even though it was against all hospital rules and she knew it. Finally, the doctors relented. I knew and maybe Maureen did too that her prognosis wasn't good and the doctors knew how much this meant to her.

When the day came, Maureen got out of bed and slowly put herself together. She put on underwear and pants and a sweater even though everything was swollen and tender. I put on her shoes. She sat in front of the hospital mirror and covered her yellow skin with makeup. She drew on eyebrows and glued on eyelashes. Her hands shook and she waited between each step to get her breath back. She couldn't wear a wig, so she wrapped a scarf around her head and made sure you couldn't see any of her scalp. Last she put on a surgical mask and said, "I'm ready, Bill. Let's go see the boys."

I helped her stand and get in the car, and we drove 45 minutes to the school. When we got to the school auditorium, Maureen walked in like she did this every day. I had called the Cranford Elementary School ahead of time and explained to them what was going on, so they would understand the severity of the situation. Ryan's whole class had written letters to Maureen telling her to get better and keep smiling, the way kids do.

The night of the concert one of the teachers met me at a side door. After Maureen was out of the car, the teacher walked ahead of us, leading us to the auditorium. They had a chair saved for Maureen right at the back. She sat forward on her chair and kind of leaned out into the aisle so Erik would be sure to see her. When he walked on stage, his eyes went right to her, not even searching the crowd. It was like they had a secret code. Maureen didn't cry that night, but I did. Ryan stood up from about the fourth row back and waved. That's all he could do, but he kept turning around during the concert to peek at her. She put all her courage into a smile that showed like a sunrise in her eyes. The boys just couldn't get enough of her. As soon as the concert was over, I drove her right back to Hackensack Hospital. Maureen was limp and sick, but she was happy.

"I have to see my boys, Bill," she said as I helped her into bed. She repeated it two more times.

The days after the chemotherapy were counted down to day 0. On that day Maureen received the first stem cell infusion, and she received an infusion every day until the cells grafted. Maureen and all the others getting cells put back into their bodies sat in the big recliner chairs again. This time it was more like a blood transfusion, but with additional medications and a preservative from when the stem cells were frozen. That preservative gave all the patients a horrible taste in their mouth. I learned fast to have Life Savers or lemon drops ready.

The second phase had been just as devastating as the first. But now Maureen had reached the reason for enduring all the pain. The stem cells could now take over. Stem cell grafting is when new bone marrow cells start to work and make new blood cells. The doctors told us it could take almost two weeks before they would know if new cells were working. Every day they weighed Maureen, and took her blood pressure and temperature. She had blood and platelet transfusions also every day which included antibiotics, electrolyte supplements and medication to help with the nausea. The whole process took about six hours. She had shots of Neupogen to help the new cells grow. Maureen was wiped out.

I stayed with her as much as I possibly could, but once in a while a nurse or a doctor told me to go for a walk or get a cup of coffee. I learned every one's name and new every inch of that wing. The nurses nicknamed me the mayor, because I helped the other families too. If one of the women started to throw up in the lunchroom at the same time that I was getting juice for Maureen, I'd go over and help out. I'd be catching throw up from this lady or throw up from that lady. It didn't matter. Everybody's outfit was a robe and a throw-up bucket—that's what we brought back and forth from our quarantine rooms to the hospital every day.

I took care of people that weren't patients too, other women's friends and even their spouses. I can't tell you how many times I held people that were crying. I was acting strong while Maureen was in the other room. But a lot of times I was so upset, I climbed the staircase and sat on the top of the stairwell and cried. I didn't want Maureen to see me crying, so the stairwell was my spot. My home was the chair beside her bed. Weeks went by and I hardly slept; I didn't' want to miss anything. I had to stay awake. Only those times when the morphine made her sleep did I head up to the top floor of the stairwell. The nurses knew where to find me.

Maureen spent Thanksgiving 1997 in a hospital bed. I brought Erik and Ryan in to have some kind of holiday. Maureen looked awful; her skin was yellowish-gray, her hair was gone and her stomach, hands and legs were bloated. She did her best to be cheerful, but she didn't have the strength.

Maureen's Journal

11/20/97 Friday The hospital & staff was <u>very</u> organized. A therapist came every day to exercise & walk me. Everyday I showered, ate pretty good. Bill <u>never</u> left. Slept (or attempted to) every night there. Friday night everything stopped, but kept the bladder catheter in until Sunday morning.

11/21/97 Evening found traces of blood in urine, so fluid intake was increased. That night I was uncomfortable.

11/23/97 Was released from hospital & went to Royal Crown Hotel. Slept a lot until next week. Blood counts were all down low & had no energy. Lots of stomach pain & gas. Enough gas to get me to California & back. My insides were totally tore up. Food & nausea. Could not keep anything down. Felt awful.

11/23/97 Monday. Went to the clinic at 9 a.m. Got my stem cells back. Got sick after that. Stayed until 5 p.m. Everyday went to clinic & sat with 6 other women. Transfusion or just fluids. Sunday & Saturday & Thanksgiving went to hospital. Got a rash so they kept me away from the group for a few days. The boys came Thanksgiving, but I slept almost all the time. Ryan left a note to see if I was having nice dreams. My boys are really 2 people I'm very proud of. I love them more than they know. Someday good things will come to them for all this. I was able to come <u>HOME</u> Dec. 3. I was happy & scared. I was also weak & so tired & sick. Went to GP daily for blood test.

Maureen and I waited for the stem cells to graft and reproduce so the blood counts would rise. As soon as the doctors decided that her stem cells had engrafted and she was growing her own red and white blood cells and platelets, Maureen had her wig on. She wanted to get home and see the boys. The stem cell chemotherapy reduced all the swelling and hardness of her left breast so that it now looked and felt normal. We knew it would take six to twelve months before Maureen had normal blood counts, but we both had hope.

When Maureen got home after all the stages of stem cell therapy, she went to Dr. Mullen's office every day to get blood drawn. Maureen wasn't allowed in the local hospital, because she had no immune system, and whenever the boys came into the house, they had to go in through the basement and scrub up with Lysol before they could see their Mom. I followed them, washing the door, the stairs, the doorknobs, the countertops, the sink faucets and the flusher on the toilets. I followed them everywhere with disinfectants. It wasn't life as we had known it, but we had Maureen back. We started looking forward and thinking things might be o.k.

The report from Hackensack was great. The tumor had shrunk, Maureen was in good shape for surgery, and she was getting enough platelets. Everything was going as planned. Now she could proceed with the mastectomy. It was a funny thing to look forward to in the new year, but Maureen hooked her life on those new days and pulled herself toward them. She was going to make it.

Mastectomy planned
Medical Record 12/3/97
Plan left mastectomy in January

Medical Record 12/4/97
Phone call: Spoke with doctor from Hackensack.
Updated on Mrs. Thiel's care

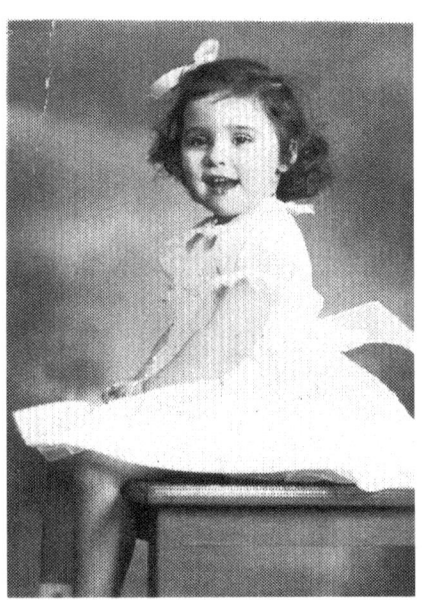

Maureen Elizabeth Davies born February 3, 1955

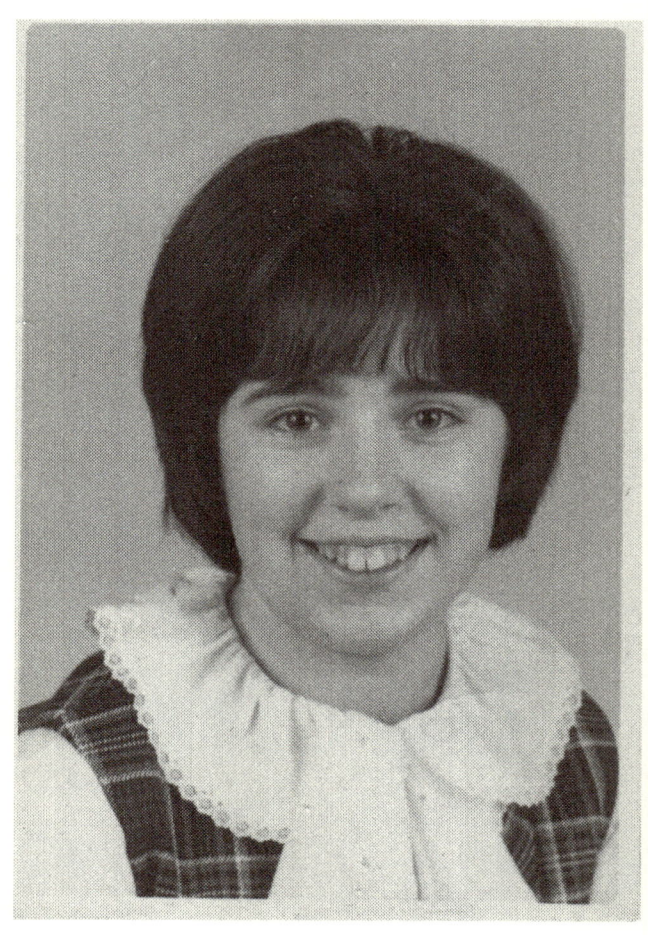

Maureen in Junior High School

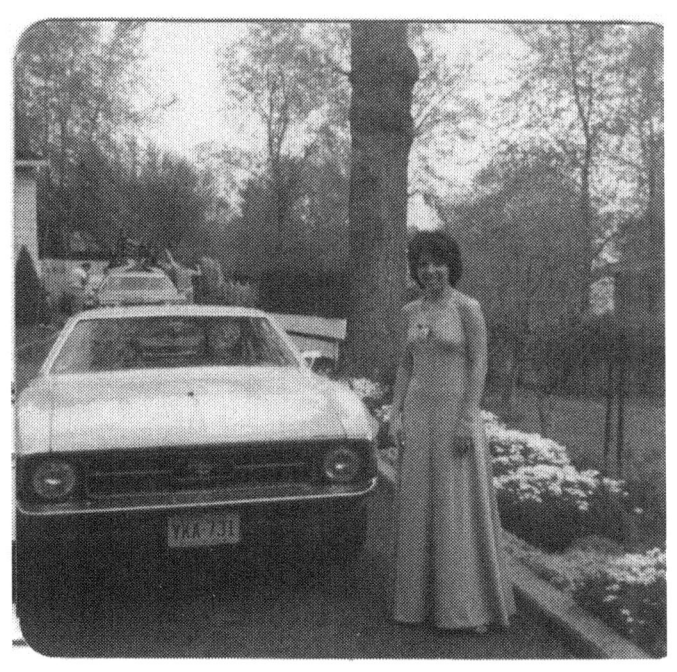

Maureen going to the prom, 1973

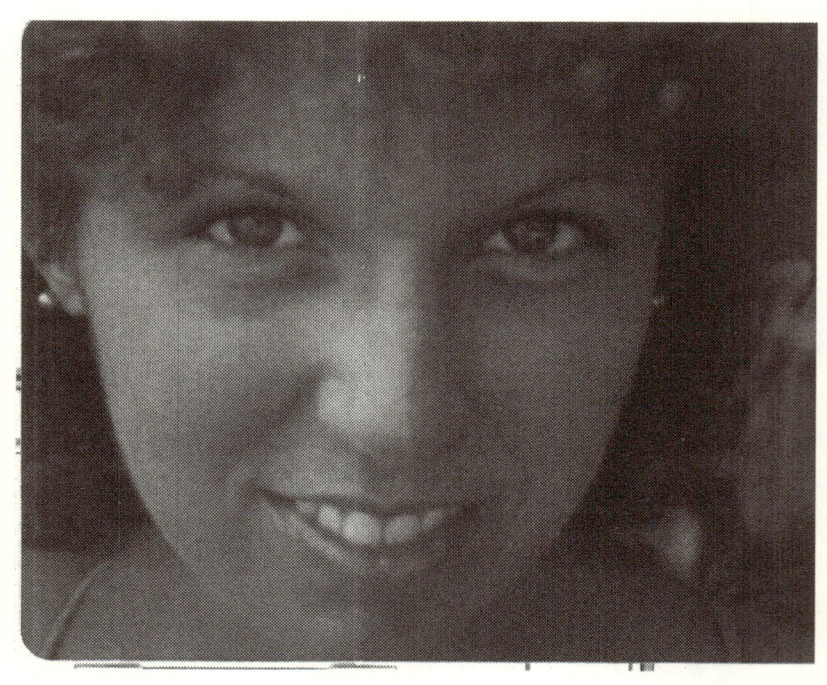

Maureen at 26

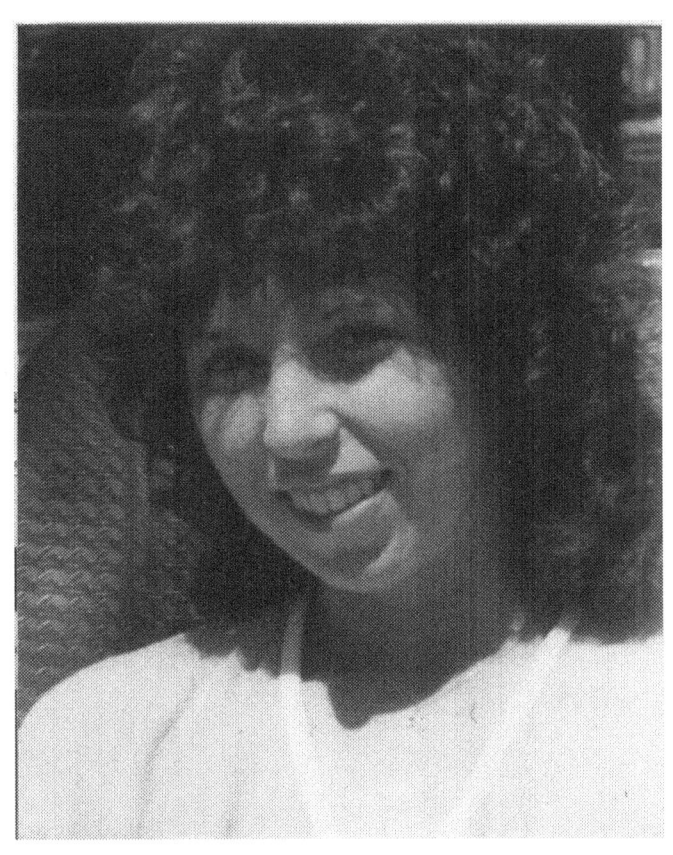

Maureen at 28

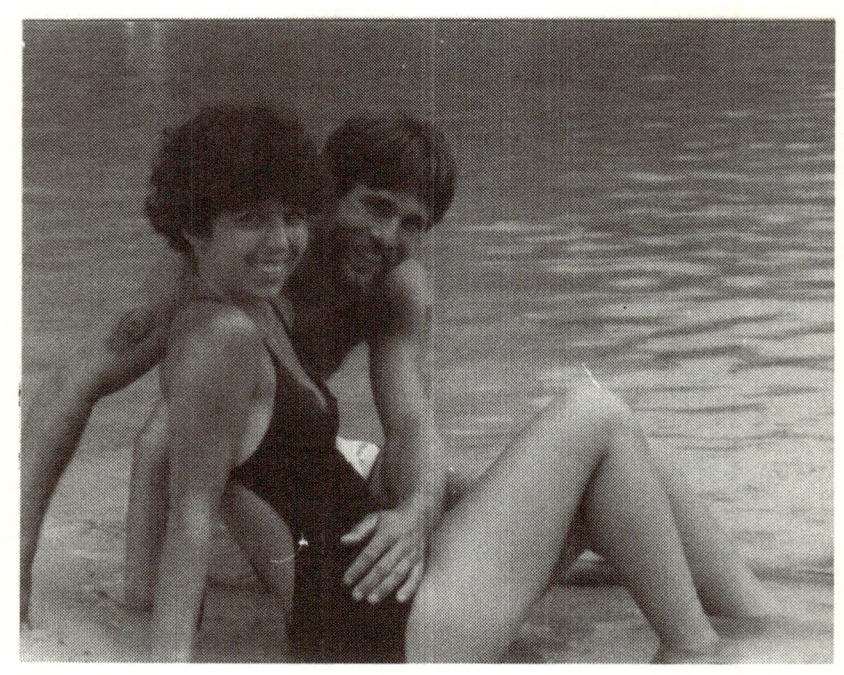

Maureen and Bill at Sand Key Beach, Florida

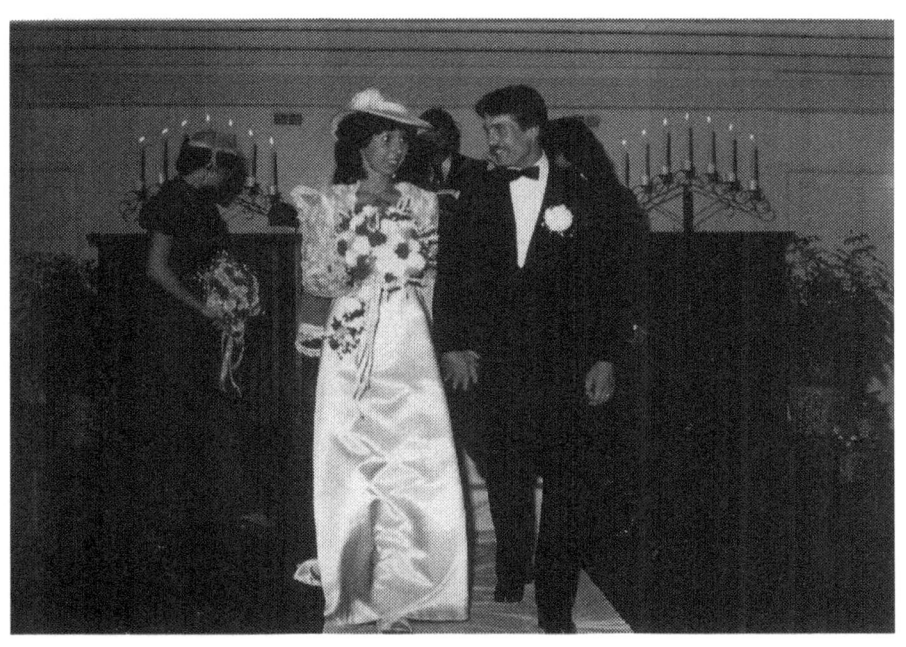

Mr. and Mrs. William Thiel, Florida 1984

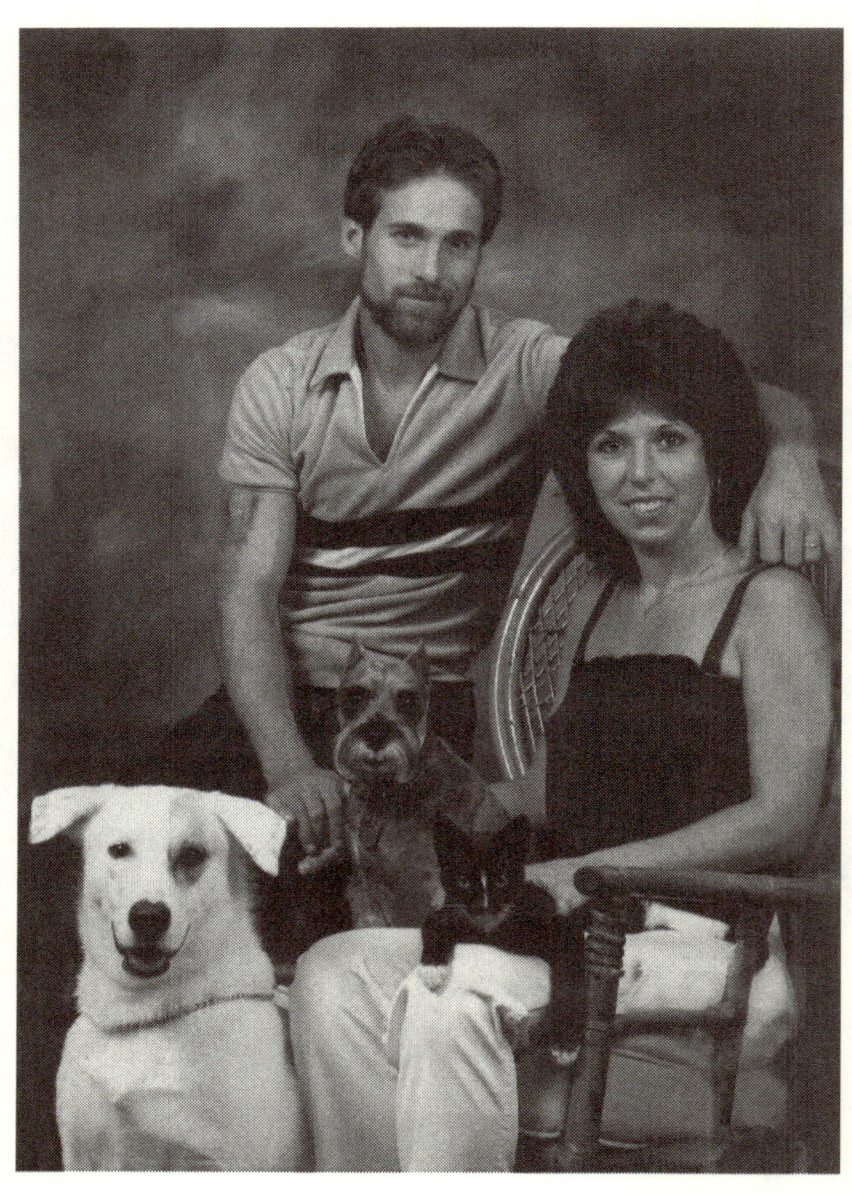

Maureen, Bill, Heidi, Kitty and Sheba 1985

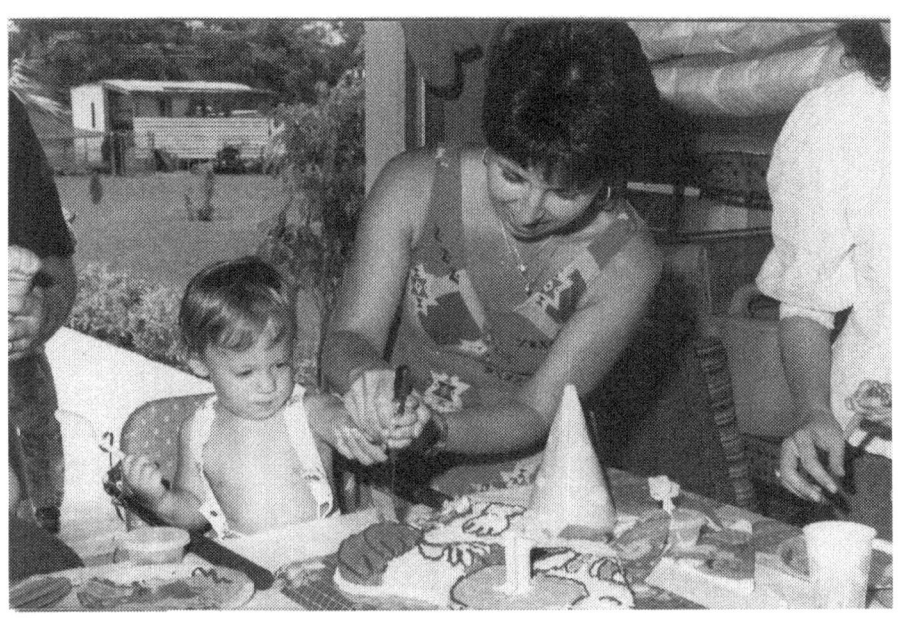

Maureen with Erik on his first birthday

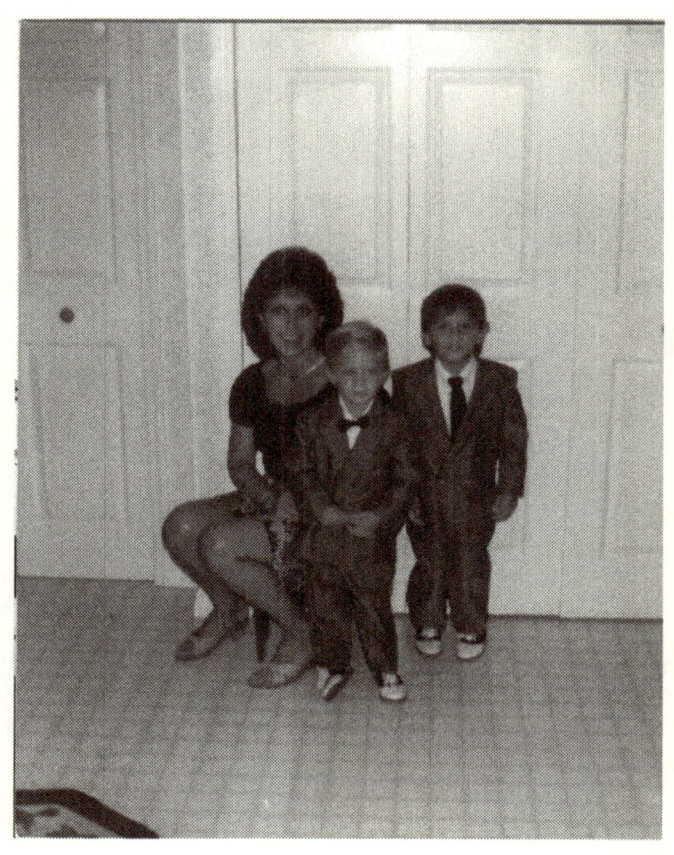

Maureen with Erik and Ryan

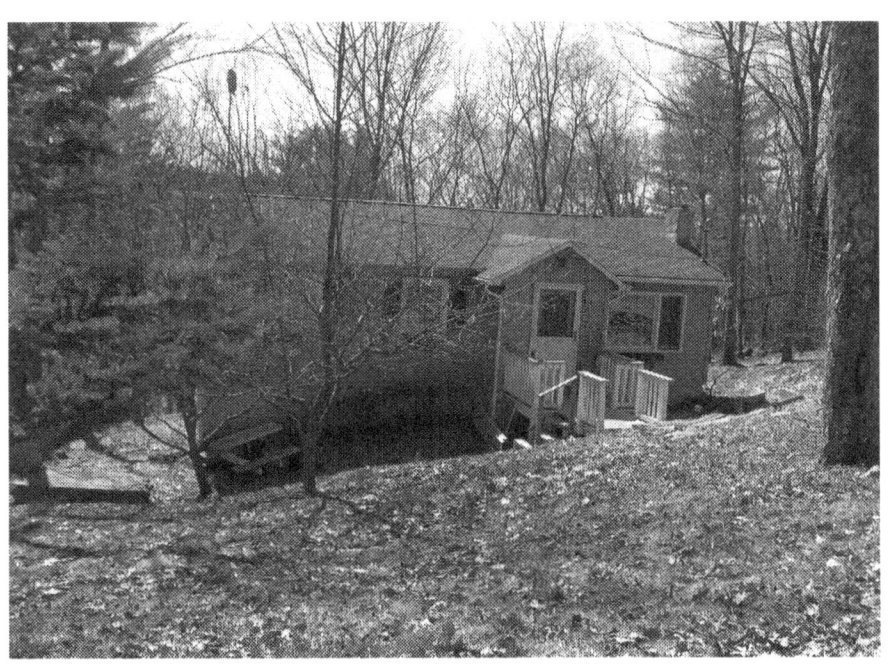

The house in Bushkill, PA

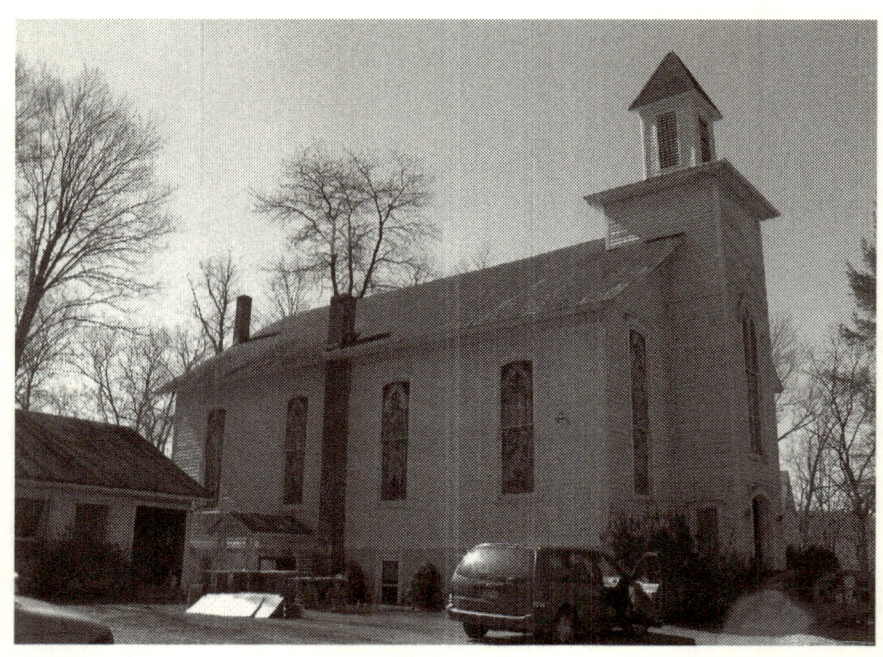

The Reformed Church of Bushkill, PA

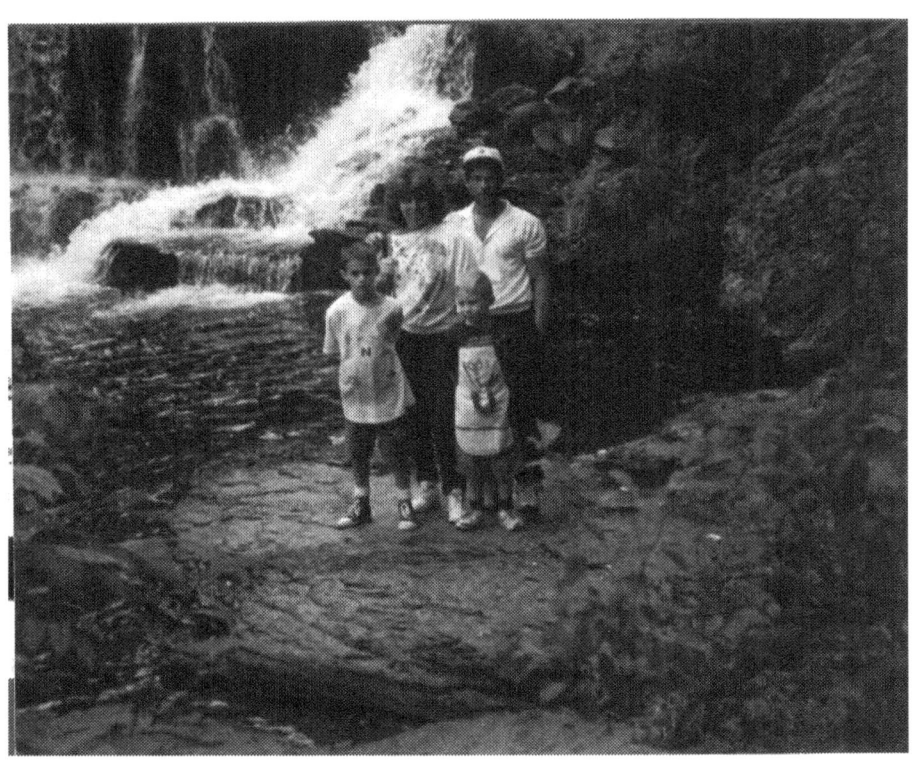

Maureen, Bill, Erik and Ryan at Watkins Glen, NY

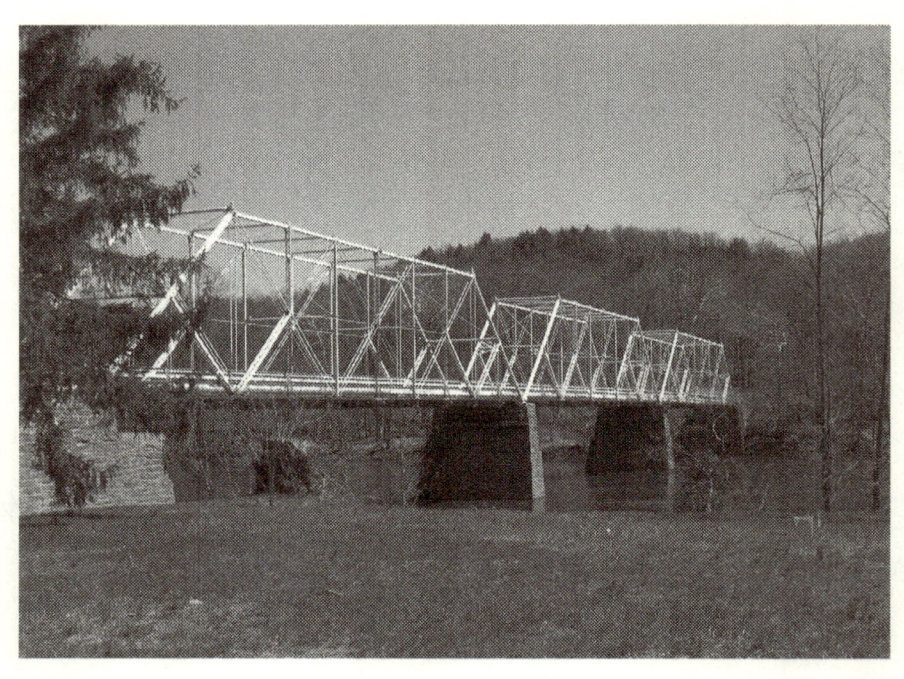

Dingmans Bridge, Delaware National Park

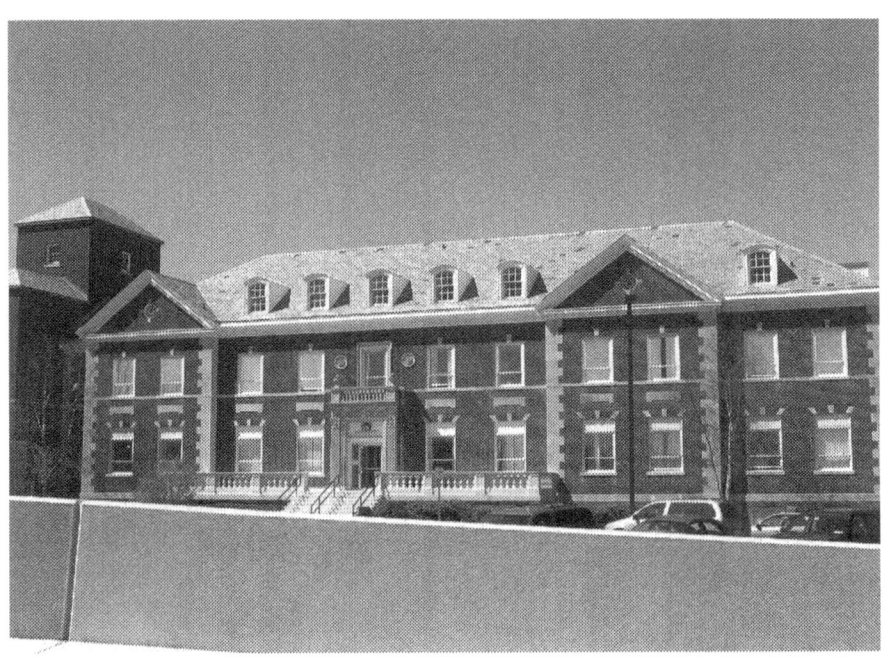

Newton Memorial Hospital

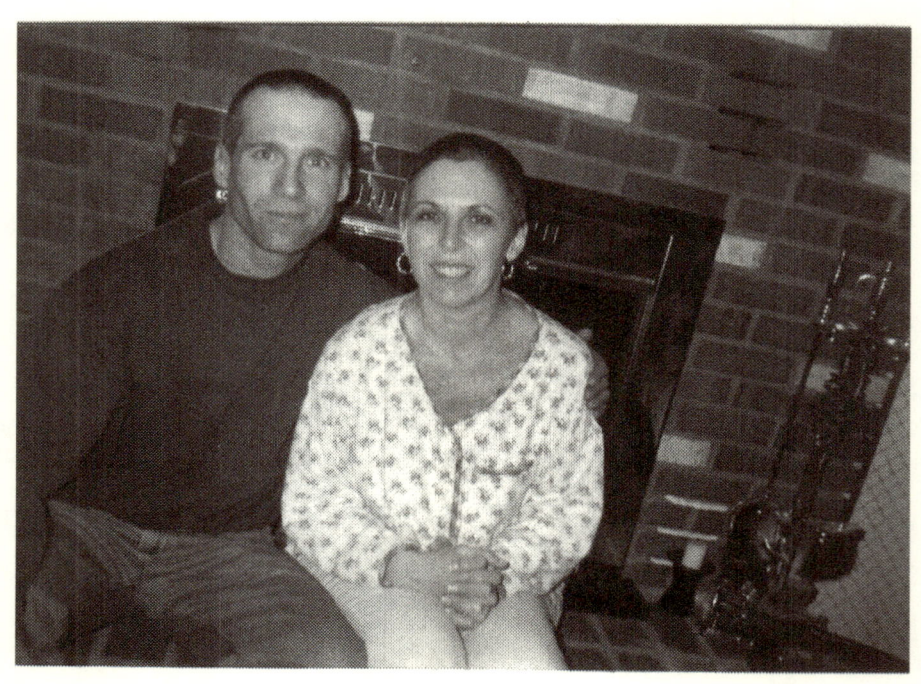

Maureen and Bill with shaved heads during first chemotherapy

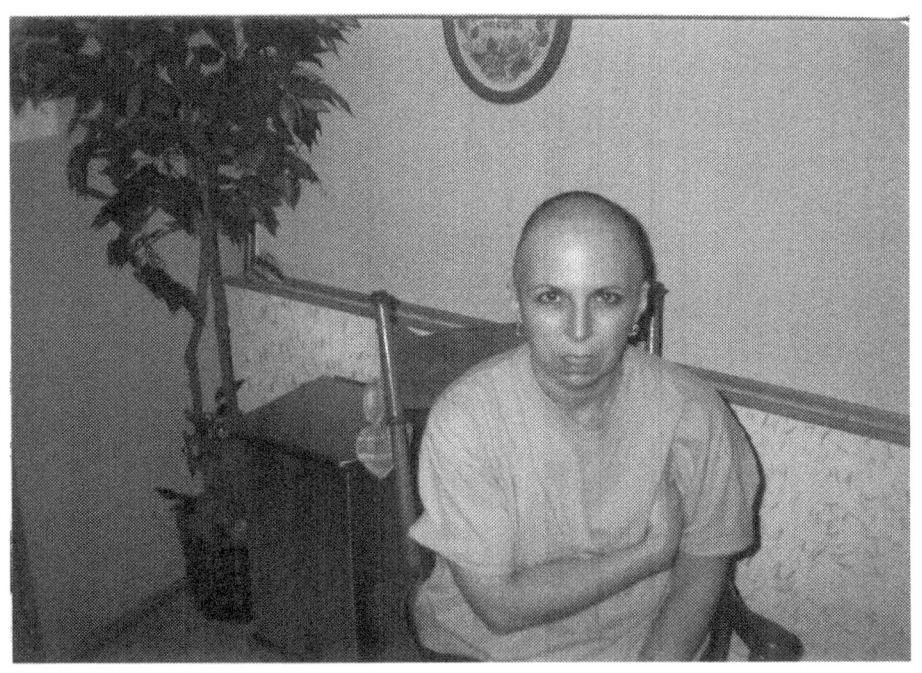

Maureen during stem cell therapy at Hackensack, NJ

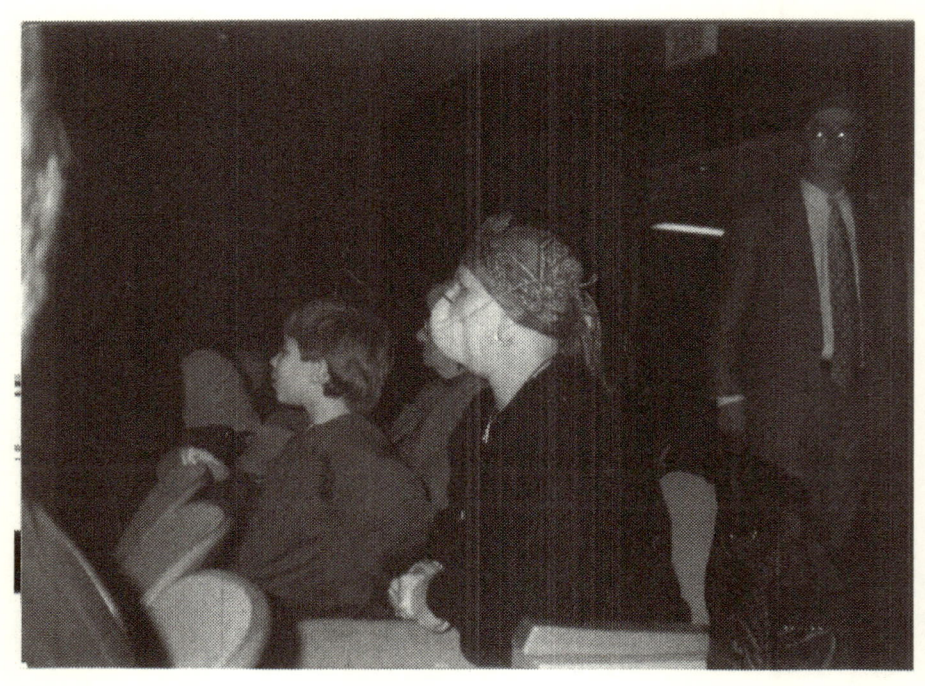

Maureen attending Erik's concert while undergoing stem cell therapy

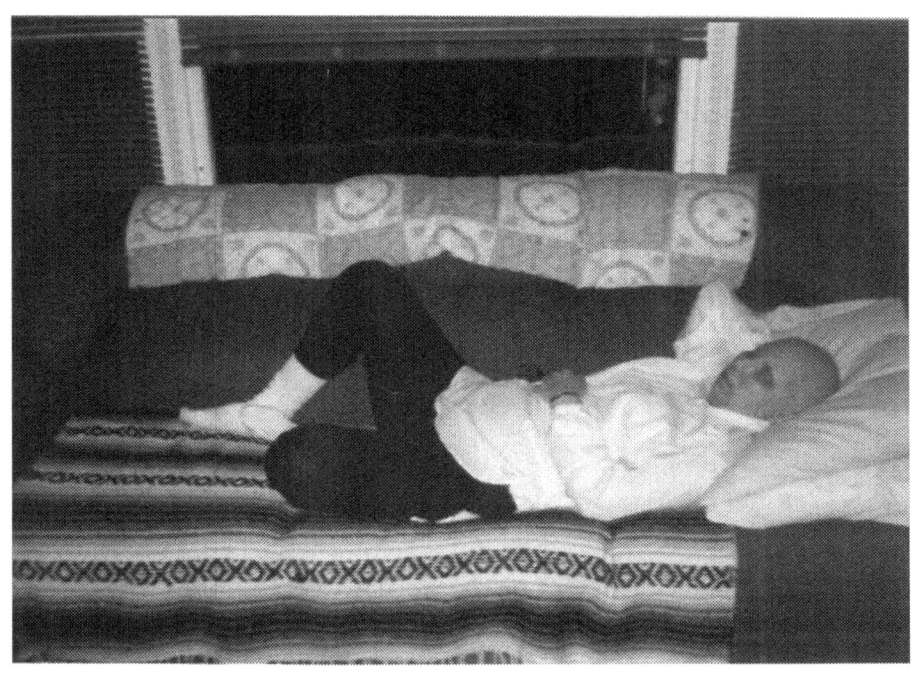

Maureen at home in Bushkill after stem cell therapy

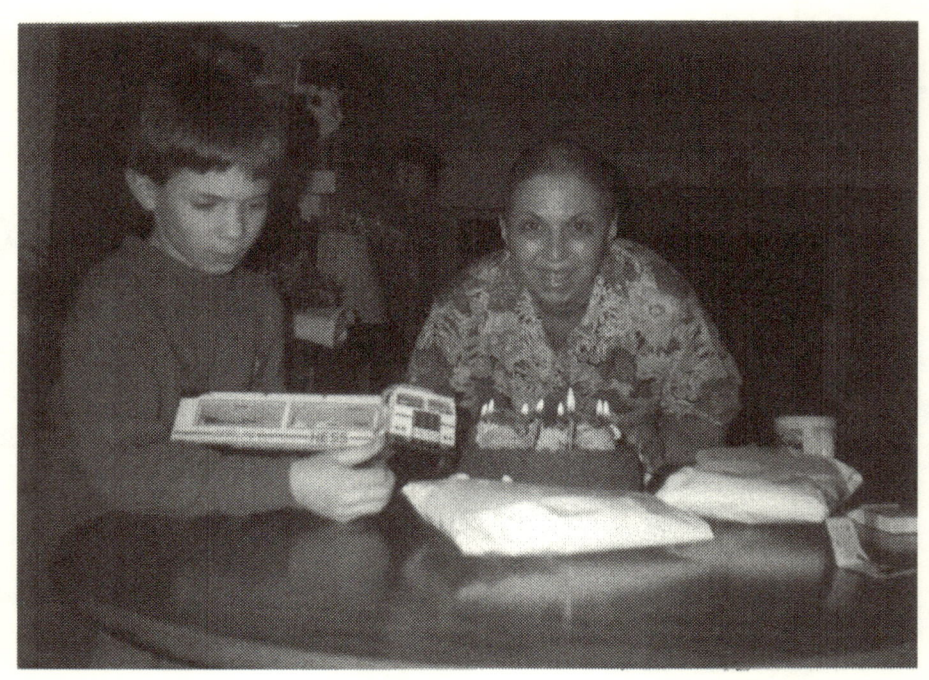

Maureen giving Ryan his 10th birthday party

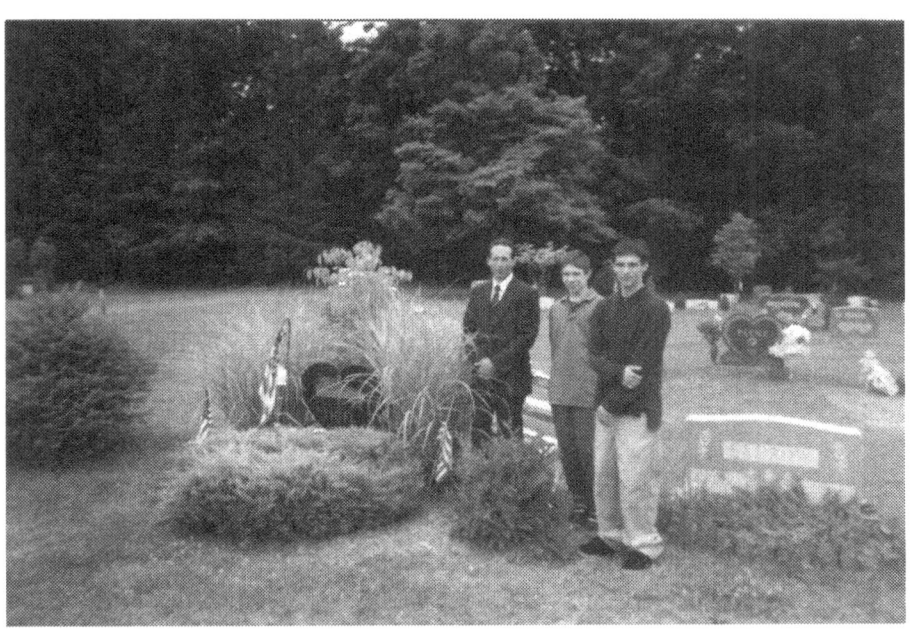

Bill, Erik and Ryan at Maureen's grave, 2004

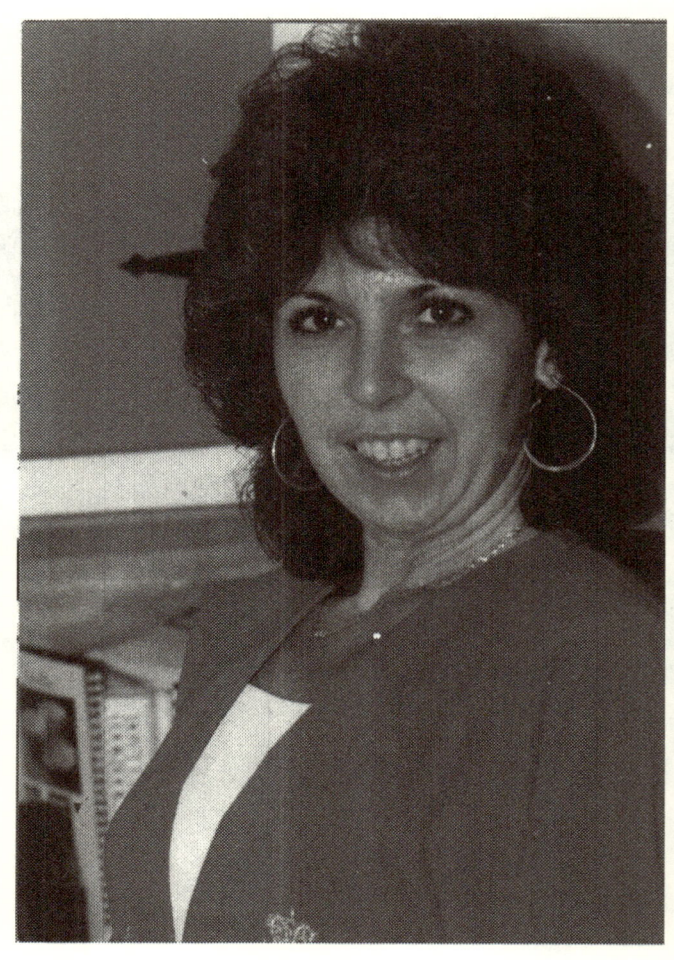

Maureen Elizabeth Thiel 3/3/55–5/16/98

Chapter Five

A Promise

We left the Hackensack Medical Center on December third and went to see the surgeon to plan the mastectomy for some time in January.

On our way home, Maureen was pretty quiet, but I could see her taking in everything as we drove.

Left mastectomy scheduled
Medical Record 12/3/97
Office Visit
Plan Left mastectomy in January.

"Everything looks new," she said.

All the leaves were long gone off the trees and it was one of those early December days that never really let the sun in. Everything looked hunched and stiff.

"Yeah, it feels good to be out." I knew what she meant. This was her chance to take her life back, to start again from before that scream had pulled everything away. She wasn't going to give an inch.

Even though we were out of Hackensack, we still had to go back to Newton Memorial everyday to check on her blood counts and get transfusions. It was our job now, our daily routine.

Maureen's blood counts were still nowhere near a healthy range. The Hemoglobin (Hgb) should be at 12.5 to 15 grams per deciliter and she was only at 9.1. Maureen's body was hanging on, struggling to make it. Maureen tried to do the things that made up the life she wanted to live. I Stayed very close and watched her all the time. I puttered around with fix-up chores so she wouldn't know I was keeping an eye on her.

Transfuse platelets
Medical Record 12/9/97
Office Notes
WBC 6.0
Hgb is 9.1
platelets are 34K.
Plan to transfuse platelets today.

I watched her one Tuesday morning, after the boys left for school. She sat at the kitchen table and began a project for the Church just the way she always did. Small pots of tempera paints were lined up in front of her. The paintbrush rested in the curve of her fingers like it was part of her hand. She had capable hands that liked to be busy. She set balsa wood pieces on a newspaper spread flat. The glue was dry, so the flat, cutout pieces held together in a spiky circle. On top of these were more balsa wood shapes, cut like holly leaves. It was a wreath for the church bazaar. She was ready to paint the leaves a deep, shiny blue/green. She had learned to begin with the green and add an overlay of blue to give the right effect, she said. Later, she would go back and place several sets of red beads in place for berries. The final touch was a green and red plaid bow. It was her Welsh signature.

She dipped the brush into the pot holding the green paint and began to stroke the paint onto a wooden leaf. Her hand held steady for a while, but on the fourth trip from the paint pot to the leaf, she faltered. A slight vibration began in her wrist then spread along her fingers until the brush jittered up and down, until gripping was impossible, until the paint dripped and splashed a jagged line across the leaf like a canker worm tunneling across the veins. Maureen dropped the brush onto the newspaper, not caring that it might dry there and stick to the newsprint. Not caring that she had promised the wreath for Saturday. She pushed herself away from the table and went to the couch. She pulled the afghan around her and curled into herself, her eyes dry and hollow as she watched the snow slant down through the bare apple trees. I waited until she fell asleep, then I put the lids back on the paints and washed out her brush.

After the transfusions, Maureen's energy perked up a little and her spirits rose. But the trips to the hospitals took a lot out of her. Riding in the car made her dizzy and weak, and it took hours for the transfusions. She had to do it though, because the platelets are the cells that help the blood clot. Any bleeding would be hard to stop, and if the number of platelets dropped too low, she could bleed from her nose or rectum. That was one of the daily realities she lived with.

Transfuse platelets
Medical Record 12/9/97
Newton Memorial Hospital
Platelet transfusion for thrombocytopenia

Even so, Maureen insisted on doing all the housework right up until she couldn't do anything. She wasn't a martyr, she was just hell bent on keeping things as normal as possible. She ran the vacuum and got the kids off to school. They were old enough to help out, but Maureen needed to be their mom. She could have had help from neighbors and people from the church too, but she kept people away so they wouldn't see her so sick. That was why she took such care to have the right wig and the right makeup. How many people would care at that point? Maureen hated anyone feeling sorry for her.

Maureen's Journal

12/8/97 Had a transfusion I believe 12/8 or 12/9.

12/10/97 Had the chest catheter removed at Morristown. Felt good to get that out & be able to have a shower without being covered in plastic. Counts were doing better, so saw GP less & less per week. Bill was able to go back to work. I still have to stay away from groups of people, but life is getting better & I'm feeling stronger.

Getting one of the catheters out was a huge relief and made us both feel like we were starting to move in a better direction. The platelet count was improving, too. The real good news came a few days later.

Removed catheter
Medical Record 12/10/97
Morristown Memorial Hospital
Right chest wall Perma-cath removed

Medical Record 12/11/97
Office Visit
Comes in for a blood count.
White count is 5.3 with a platelet count of 89K

The stem cells were working. The cancer cells that had been killed in the chemotherapy were being replaced with new, healthy ones. Maureen made it through stem cell therapy and we were home. Home with the boys, just the four of us again, being the family we always were. Maureen still wasn't up to decorating the house for the holidays, so the boys and I put up a tree and tried to make the house look the way it did when Maureen did it. Maureen directed us from the couch. When I asked her how many strings of lights she wanted, I didn't get an answer. She had nodded off to sleep.

Bone scan
Medical Record 12/15/97
Newton Memorial Hospital
Whole Body Bone Scan:
'an overall substantial improvement in the bony metastasis.'

The next day, Maureen sat watching the lights twinkle when there was a knock on the door.

"Who is it?" Maureen wanted to know.

Then she heard the voices. She started to get up but remembered she couldn't have company. It was a group from the church wanting to sing Christmas carols for her. Maureen sat back down, trying not to look disappointed, but I knew she wanted to see somebody other than me. Snow came down in slow, big flakes and the light had faded from the day. Maureen pulled the afghan over her then went very still. She got up and walked to the window. Out on our little front lawn twelve people were singing. "Oh, come all ye faithful, joyful and triumphant ... "

Maureen put her hand to the window and sang along. They sang "Silver Bells" and "Silent Night." Before they turned to go, Maureen blew them a kiss. She only let them see her smiles.

All that December I took Maureen back to the hospital for platelet transfusions. I called ahead and let them know we were coming because Maureen had no immune system so she couldn't sit in a waiting room or walk down a hallway with other people. We developed a routine for arriving at the hospital: I'd go in and tell the nurses we were waiting, then I'd go back out and sit with Maureen in the car. I kept the car running, but Maureen was always cold. She had nothing in her to keep her warm. I piled blankets on her, but sometimes we waited a long time for a clear room, and I couldn't leave the car running all that time. When a room finally opened, a nurse met us at the door. She would have cleared the hallway and another nurse would be on the elevator ready to whip Maureen right into a room. It was a very lonely time; all these procedures were alienating, and Maureen was embarrassed at the way she looked and how weak she had become. Her platelet counts were still dropping and her blood wouldn't clot. I never told her how many panties I threw away because she was bleeding so much.

Maureen's Journal

12/20/97 Christmas we went to Cranford to my Mom's. The boys were still there going to school until Dec. 23.

The boys were doing the best they could. All the nurses and doctors knew them too by now, especially at Newton Memorial. One nurse, I think his name was Ken entertained Erik and Ryan by blowing up a latex glove and putting it on his head. He taught the boys how to put a rubber band around the spray nozzle on a sink so that when someone turned it on, they got sprayed. They did that at Katheryn's house and got into some trouble. They were just trying to be kids.

Maureen's Journal

12/26/97 Stayed until Christmas afternoon. I was feeling tired & very warm. My feet swelled up & I couldn't wait to come home. The boys returned home too. Their time at Ma's wasn't all fun & games. They had hard times too. No school until Jan. 5. I rested a lot. Saw GP. Told him about my feet swelling, but he says not to worry with what I went through.

We spent that Christmas with our families even though I still traveled with a throw up bucket and Maureen had her head wrapped in a bandanna. During the Christmas season, Maureen and I always had a glass of eggnog with rum and cinnamon each night before we went to bed. That Christmas, Maureen poured me a cup of eggnog and put in a little rum. She poured herself a glass of juice and we clinked glasses. "Here's to hope," she said. I said it back to her, but I was holding my breath for the stem cells to fully graft. Maureen was full of hope. Everything in her said, "We're gonna beat this." The stem cell therapy was supposed to give her a year or two of time until technology could catch up. Or maybe it would wipe out the cancer all together.

Soon it was New Year's Eve 1997. All Maureen wanted to do was make it into the next year, to 1998. She prayed to have New Years with the boys, and then everything would get better. She wanted to put 1997 behind her, and she was optimistic that the stem cell treatment was the silver bullet. She had made it through, and her breast was no longer hard from the tumor. The cancer was still there, but she was fighting it. In all this time, Maureen never heard the word 'remission'. It must be a great word to hear. I never heard it, so I can't say what it's like.

Maureen's fighting got her to New Year's Eve. The boys wanted to see *Titanic*, and so did she. It had just debuted, and the local movie theater had a special New Year's showing that started at 11:00 p.m. That way, when *Titanic* was over it would be New Years Day, 1998. Maureen thought it was a great way to celebrate the New Year with the boys. That afternoon I was making sandwiches for myself and the boys and I heard, "Bill, come here."

Maureen was in the bathroom.

"Oh, shit." I ran this time.

She said, "Feel this."

I felt her breast. The cancer had come back. Her breast had hardened up again only fifteen days after the most powerful chemotherapy she could have. If you can imagine a candle burning and melting slowly, then suddenly dissolving, all melted down, that's what Maureen felt. That's what I felt too. Devastated isn't even close to the right word.

I said, "Let's call the doctors. Let's get you over there."

"No," she said, "I told Erik and Ryan we're going to see *Titanic* tonight, and we're going. If I call the doctor, they're going to put me in the hospital."

"Are you sure?"

"Yes."

I wasn't going to argue with her. I supported her one hundred percent, I had no right to question that she wanted to spend that night with the boys.

That day was a numb day. She didn't let the boys know anything about the cancer coming back; they were only nine and eleven. We went to the cinema and watched *Titanic*. To this day, I can't listen to the song from that movie. It's a great story and a great movie, but when the movie ended, confetti came down like a Happy New Year party with music. Everyone was so happy and holding each other, but Maureen and I stood there crying, holding each other because we knew it was our last New Year's together. Neither one of us said anything. The boys smiled at us, thinking "Oh, Mom and Dad are happy. They really love each other." Those things were true. We loved each other, but we knew.

Maureen's Journal

1/2/98 Went back to GP. I'm a bit nervous. The breast seems to be getting firm again. GP agrees. He's calling surgeon. Surgeon called. Tomorrow, I'm going to Morristown to get breast removed. 7:30 a.m.

The very next day, Maureen called the doctor and immediately went in to the hospital. The doctors had planned on a mastectomy after her stem cell anyway to get rid of this cancer. This was the best plan.

Cancer reemerges in left breast
Medical Record 01/02/98
Office Visit
c/o left breast larger and more firm 'The left breast is definitely more firm ... disturbingly on the right side there may be a little bit of firmness in a crescent shaped configuration in the upper portion of the right breast ... referral to surgeon for mastectomy ... have also put in a call to oncologist.

Maureen knew in her mind she was going have this mastectomy, but now it wasn't in the future. She had an emergency, radical mastectomy, immediately at the beginning of January.

Infiltrating. Extending. Invading. That was the results from all the tests and the scans. The cancer had spread. Maureen was so tired from the stem cell process, and the surgery wiped her out. But it was this news that took every bit of wind out of her sails.

Left mastectomy
Medical Record 01/03/98
Morristown Memorial Hospital
Left Modified Radical Mastectomy & Interpectoral lymph node dissection. Path Report: 'infiltrating, poorly differentiated carcinoma extension into reticular dermis ... extending into superficial portion of attached skeletal muscle ... invading numerous lymphatic and vascular spaces involving soft tissue less than 1 mm from deep resection margin.'

Maureen's Journal

1/3/98 Don't remember being in recovery, but in room I'm lost & can't figure out what has happened to me. Before I'm awake, my Mom & sister are there. Too much confusion. I'm tired & I hurt.

1/4/98 Sunday. I feel a bit better, but I'm depressed. Found more cancer in the breast. Can't believe the stem cell didn't kill it. I need radiation now. I'm running out of treatments. I hope God has a miracle in his plans for me. The church has been wonderful. Carol Scoble has planned everything. Everyday dinner comes to the house. The minister, Steve Sayer, came to hospital Sat. & Sun. Just pray for me. There's so much living I still have to do!

That was the last entry in Maureen's journal. She didn't have the energy or the heart to put anymore of her thoughts down on paper. The boys came with me as much as they could to visit Maureen in the hospital. They wanted to see their mom and make her happy, but often it was too hard for them. Erik shot basketballs outside the hospital even when it was freezing, just to stay away from the room. Maureen was too upset for him to bear. As Maureen got weaker, she and I got more closed in our ability to let other people share our pain. Part of that was biological and medical. There were all sorts of reasons for limiting contact, because Maureen's immune system was gone. But some of it was emotional as well. We treasured our time together, and we had always been complete in each other. That feeling grew as she became more ill.

Maureen had the mastectomy just as planned, but it was another battle to face after all she'd been through. I don't know how any woman deals with losing a breast. Maureen knew this had to happen and even looked forward to it in a way, but when it finally did happen, something inside her crumpled. I didn't care if my wife had one breast or no breasts. I didn't marry her for her breasts; I married her for her heart.

Surgery complete; more questions
Medical Record 01/05/98
Discharged from Morristown Memorial Hospital

Medical Record 01/05/98
Office Records
Phone call from Bill Thiel: Maureen feels like there is something in her throat.
Instructed by doctor that this is probably post intubation. 'They are coming in a couple of days to discuss experimental therapy options.'

Once Maureen had the mastectomy, there was another set of bandages and concerns to work with every day. I had to be careful every time I bathed her. The way I wrapped her with the double Quinton was one way, the way I wrapped the surgical area after the mastectomy was a different way. The surgery gave us both a little relief. I guess we both thought, "Well, the tumor's gone now." We always tried to see the glass as half full, never half empty. But I felt so sad for Maureen. It was like seeing something beautiful taken apart piece by piece, nothing ever given, just constant taking away.

At this point the boys were home alone much of the time. I know Maureen's illness hurt them the worst. It just went from Maureen always being there to not ever being there. That was the biggest change. Erik sat in his room, and the house got very messy. Because Maureen and I were hardly ever home, Erik and Ryan started fighting. Sometimes they fixed their own dinner, but a lot of times they went to a friend's house. As much as the neighbors could, they kept the boys with them either at their houses or at the clubhouse and pool. But it was weird for the boys. They didn't want to think it was happening to them. One night Maureen and I came home from the hospital and Erik told me they'd just eaten chocolate for dinner.

CAT scan
Medical Records 01/09/98
Office Visit Comes in today for a blood count.
She is on her way to see surgeon.
CT scans of the chest, abdomen and pelvis were ordered.

Maureen was ready to start radiation. It's what they do right after a mastectomy. Every day she saw Doctor Godard, the radiologist and Doctor Mullen. Everyday Doctor Mullen checked her and examined her other breast. After a few of these visits he told her to see the surgeon. She had an appointment to see him that day anyway.

Drain removed
Medical Record 01/09/98
Office Visit w/surgeon
One surgical drain removed

The surgeon looked Maureen over carefully and told her to come back in a week to have the other drain removed. I asked him to call Doctor Mullen, and I know they talked before we came back again.

The surgeon that did the emergency radical mastectomy took the second drain out. I asked him to examine Maureen's right breast, and after he did, he immediately did a biopsy. In less than 30 days after stem cell therapy the cancer had come back in her right breast. Maureen didn't quit. If I could match one millionth of her strength, I'd be lucky. But this news wasn't good.

On January 20th, we were all home and the boys were asleep. Maureen surprised me by getting into our bed after not sleeping in our room since the summer. I was in the living room and I heard her call.

"Bill, come here." She said.

It was a nice "Bill, come here." I didn't have to run.

I lay down next to her and I kissed her softly on her cheekbones, on her chin, on her mouth.

Right breast aspiration: suspect cancer
Medical Record 01/16/98
Fine Needle Aspiration of Right Breast Second surgical drain
removed Pathology: 'Markedly atypical cells occurring singly
and in clusters.
Highly suspicious for ductal carcinoma.'

"I want to love you the way I used to Bill," she whispered. "I want to show you everything I feel. The last time we made love was in June."

I gathered her to me as gently as I could, but when I looked down at her, huge tears were welling up under her lids. It just hurt too much.

"Every day you make love to me, Maureen." I told her, "It doesn't have to be physical."

We held each other and cried until our breathing moved back and forth together like a deep ocean that could rock us away from our sorrow.

After a long while, Maureen asked me, "Bill, will you make me a promise?"

"Of course I will."

"The first promise I want you to make is that you finish this lawsuit for me."

I was in left field, I hadn't been thinking about the lawsuit at all, just getting Maureen to wherever she needed to be. But that promise seemed easy, so I said, "Of course I will." I knew how important it was to her, because she had a story to tell. She was misdiagnosed three times. It was up to me to prove it so I could tell her story. That didn't seem difficult.

"I have a second promise," she continued. "Bill, I want you to promise to love the boys twice as much as you do now. I want you to love them once from you, and once from me."

I said, "O.K." I thought it was an easy promise at first, but when I thought about how much Maureen loved her boys, it wasn't simple at all. God I love my boys, but I tried to feel how much Maureen loved them and add my own love to it. I'd have to love my boys a million times more than I love them, to come anywhere near as much as Maureen loved them.

Finally, she said, "Bill I want you to promise me one last thing."

"Whatever you want, Maureen."

"Bill, I want you to love again."

I couldn't speak and my chest felt so tight I thought my lungs had turned to wood. "Bill, promise me that you'll love again." She took my hand and squeezed it. I took in some air, real shaky.

"What do you mean?"

"You have so much love in you. Don't let this keep you from going on in life."

I couldn't hear her words right and I didn't really know what she was telling me. I didn't know that when I said "O.K." I was agreeing to let someone else into my heart. That was the promise that made no sense to me. My heart was full with Maureen. She had planted a paradise that took all the space I had. Nothing else could ever find room to grow.

"Bill," she said, trying to get through to me. "I love you because of the love you have, not just for me, but for the boys, for our friends, for everything. Don't let that spoil. If down the road you meet someone, if you cross paths with someone, remember that you still have love left in you and give it to them. Promise?"

I nodded. Maureen knew what would be right for me. She knew me so well, she even knew that. She knew I wasn't going to make it on my own and that I would always need someone. So she made it easy for me to not feel guilty. But the words were like a bird singing a great song, but I didn't have any way to understand it. I wanted to love Maureen the way I had from the day I first saw her on Sand Key beach. My Maureen.

I kissed her with all my tears bottled up; I bowed my head and kissed her at the base of her throat and on top of her heart. I couldn't hold her all night the way I wanted, but I lay next to her listening as she moved through her dreams.

Soon after that, the radiation began. For forty-seven days, every day except Saturdays and Sundays, Maureen went for radiation after the mastectomy. They told us the radiation would tire Maureen out. That made Maureen laugh. Nothing could make her more tired than she already was. It was like watching a boxer taking punch after punch and still finding a way to get to her feet and face the next one. I know it was Erik and Ryan that she saw every time she was asked to do something that seemed impossible. She saw them when she was lying on the table getting the stem cell chemotherapy, and she saw them every day she lay there getting radiation.

Left chest radiation begins
Medical Record 01/21/98
UDVCC
(Upper Delaware Valley Cancer Center)
Begins Radiation therapy under the supervision of oncology radiologist.
47 days of treatment 5x/wk to the left chest wall and the left supraclavicular area.

The radiation team put little stars on her chest to mark the exact spots to receive radiation. Maureen always wanted a little tattoo, a little butterfly or angel on her shoulder, but she never got one. When they put the stars on her, she showed them to me and said, "Look Bill, I have my tattoos now." She managed to make a joke out of something that was so unfair.

Maureen talked to the doctors about a right mastectomy. She didn't want to wait, but she had to heal from the first surgery. She had to build up a little strength too. She slept almost all the time, and ate very little. When she was awake, she did her best to listen to Erik and Ryan's stories about school or their friends, but they couldn't help but see that her energy was gone.

Right mastectomy planned
Medical Record 01/22/98
Office Visit w/surgeon
Discussed suspicious nature of path report on needle aspi-
ration with Maureen and her husband.
They decided to proceed with the right mastectomy.

Medical Record 01/22/98
Office Notes
Phone Call w/primary care: Finally started on radiation
therapy to the left chest wall and spine area today.
Maureen wants to have a right mastectomy now, have
encouraged them to hold off right now unless she becomes
symptomatic.

Maureen didn't talk about the lawyers much, because she was so sick, but in January we had an appointment or two. One of the appointments was for a videotaped deposition for both her lawyers and the defense lawyers. Maureen took two hours to get dressed that morning. She had her nails done and she put on her make up. She had no eyebrows or eyelashes any more, so she had to paint everything on. She chose clothes that would look good on camera. Finally she fixed her wig. When she was done, you could not tell how sick she was. I knew. I could hear her breathing, and I could see her hands shaking. I knew all the tubes and needles that had been jabbed into her. But I saw determination in her eyes.

Maureen sat for over two hours and answered questions. They asked her about her health as a child, her pregnancies, her work, her understanding of self-breast exams, and her reasons for following the first three doctors' recommendations.

She never let them know how exhausted and weak she was. She made sure they understood everything she had to tell them, and she answered every question they had so they would know the truth.

Shortly after that visit, Maureen's right breast became swollen and hard. The doctors were hoping to finish the radiation treatments before any more surgery, but they couldn't wait.

Maureen had an emergency right mastectomy. The cancer had moved into the lymph nodes and the tissue surrounding them on the right side of her body. She came out of that surgery and read the sadness on my face. "I'm just a little bit lighter, Bill." I don't have any words for Maureen's courage.

Right mastectomy
Medical Record 01/30/98
Admission to Morristown Memorial Hospital
Right modified radical mastectomy with pectoralis minor.
Pathology report:
'infiltrating ductal carcinoma with extensive lymphatic vascular invasion … metastasis to 2/2 lymph nodes with extensive infiltration of perinodal adipose tissue.'
ER/PR negative with high S-phase.

Maureen was now in considerable and constant pain. Both sides of her body had been cut up and she was trying to heal from surgery while fighting the cancer. The doctors told me the pain would get worse. Maureen wasn't taking any chemotherapy, but she was still getting radiation. They gave her three prescriptions, all narcotics, for pain: Darvocet was for the 'mild to moderate pain,' Percocet was for the 'moderate to moderately severe' pain, and MS-Contin was for 'moderate to severe' pain. MS-Contin contains morphine. Keeping track of Maureen's pain medication was the next thing I added to my list of care-taking responsibilities.

Left hospital; Pain medication increased
Medical Record 02/02/98
Discharge from Morristown Memorial Hospital

Medical Record 02/09/98
Office Notes

'She is taking multiple doses of Darvocet for the pain in
the right shoulder and right arm. Percocet prescription
was refilled … in addition MS-Contin was prescribed.'
A suggestion was made to the husband to speak with
Hospice for counseling for the children.

The doctors and nurses told me it was time to let Hospice help. I didn't want
to, because I knew Hospice meant the end. I couldn't do it. I was taking care of
Maureen. That was my job and I didn't want anyone taking that away from me.

After the right mastectomy, on the follow up visit to Dr. Mullen, Maureen
asked him straight out how much time she had. "Three months," he said. Neither
of us said one word on the way home in the car. What do you talk about? What
do you say after someone has told you that?

Maureen went through four weeks of healing, and she still had to go to the
hospital every day for blood counts and transfusions. Maureen also started the
radiation on her right chest. The results of the lab work came in on the fax
machine at Steve Willands where I still tried to put in some time. We picked
them up on our way to Newton Memorial Hospital. Back then, Newton
Memorial wasn't set up for these daily transfusions. We would arrive at seven a.m.
and sometimes wouldn't get home until eight p.m., because we had to wait. A lot
of that has changed, and now patients don't have to wait. I like to think Maureen
had something to do with that. That was our life during February, transfusions
and more bone scans. The scans showed more cancer growth.

Right chest radiation begins
Medical Record 02/24/98
Upper Delaware Valley Cancer Center
Begins radiation treatment to the right chest wall and
supraclavicular area
36 day so treatment 5x/week.

The cumulative effect of the chemotherapy and radiation put Maureen into
full menopause. It was like watching a car going down the road at fifty or sixty
miles an hour and all of a sudden being thrown into first gear. All the symptoms
of menopause came over her like a tidal wave. She had night sweats so bad, I
changed her bedclothes four or five times a night. During the day she had hot
flashes that made her look like she had walked into a furnace. He face went red

and she gritted her teeth as wave after wave of crashing hormones collided in her. Then she went limp, like a cloth doll that's been churned up on the shore.

Bone scan; hot flashes
Medical Record 03/06/98
Office Notes
'Spoke with radiologist about the bone scan … increased uptake in the left proximal femur … x-ray ordered.
Megace 40 mg was prescribed for the "terrible, horrible hot flashes".

Maureen took hormone therapy medication to help with the menopause symptoms. She also took Megace to help treat the breast cancer. Megace is a synthetic product called progestogen that's similar to real progesterone in women's bodies. It helped, but it made her puffy from retaining fluid. They said it might help her appetite, but it never did.

The doctors had done all they could in the left chest to stop the cancer. Now they concentrated on the right mastectomy and the right chest radiation. Maureen knew I needed a distraction, something to keep my hands busy even if my mind wouldn't focus. She had always wanted a sunroom on our house, but we had never decided on a design. I got busy and started building a room for her that let in light, air and a view of the trees and flowers in our yard. I worked at night when Maureen slept or when she was with the boys or a friend. I measured, cut, hammered and painted. She told me she wanted to die in the sunroom we had planned together, so I worked.

Left chest radiation complete
Medical Record 03/09/98
Upper Delaware Valley Cancer Center
Completes 47 days of radiation treatment to the left chest wall and supraclavicular area.

Maureen had terrible headaches now. Nothing seemed to touch her pain, so we asked the doctors about it. They did a Magnetic Resonance Image or an MRI of her brain to see what was going on.

Brain metastasis; brain radiation
Medical Record 03/17/98
Office Records
Femur x-ray on the left showed sclerotic lesions only, nothing impending that is about to break.

Medical Record 03/19/98
Office Visit
MRI shows brain metastasis, multiple in the cerebellum.

Medical Record 03/19/98
Upper Delaware Valley Cancer Center
Begins radiation therapy to the brain 18 days of treatment 5x/week

I was at work, one of the rare days I could make it, when the fax machine spit out the results of Maureen's MRI. It said in black and white: brain cancer. Before I could get to my car, Maureen called. The doctor had given her the news on the phone and had already scheduled her for her first cranial radiation that day.

"I'm on my way, Maureen," I told her. "I'll be right home."

"No, Bill, there's no point. I'm just going to go."

She hung up. Just like that. I got in the car and drove back toward home and caught up to her on the road. I followed her all the way to Newton Hospital and she never knew I was right behind her until we pulled into the parking lot. There was no way I was going to let her do this by herself.

Right chest and brain radiation complete
Medical Record 04/02/98
Upper Delaware Valley Cancer Center
Completes 36 days of radiation therapy to the right chest wall and supraclavicular area.

Medical Record 04/06/98
Upper Delaware Valley Cancer Center
Completion of 18 days of radiation therapy to the brain.

Maureen needed full cranial radiation. She would never grow her hair again. The cranial radiation made her beyond tired. It fried her worse than the chest radiation, but she was still hoping because all she wanted to do was live for Erik and Ryan. I knew the hallways, the waiting area, the x-ray rooms of Newton Memorial Hospital as well as my own house. I walked so many miles in those corridors. At night there was no body there. I could go anywhere. At Newton Hospital I snuck into the records room at two or three in the morning and pulled out Maureen's x-rays. I put them up on the screen. I know I wasn't supposed to, but it didn't matter. One of the radiologists caught me one night. He looked at me for a minute and said, "I don't see you, Bill." He walked out quietly and left me to stare at Maureen's cancer.

At Easter, the church had a potluck on Maundy Thursday. Everyone was there for that. It was raining hard that morning, but Maureen wanted to be there with everyone else. She presented herself and her family just as every family did trying not to draw attention to herself. It meant everything to her to keep our normal life together.

Cele, one of the older women of the church told me that Maureen gave a lot of people courage and strength. "I just love how she comes into church with her head up. She's just beautiful." The same Sunday, Marina Cameron, the church administrator came up to me and said, "No one would know she's sick unless you look very carefully. She takes her illness in stride." Maureen did that for them, for the boys and for herself.

The church members learned to separate the announcements from the prayer requests because of us. At first they announced cookie exchanges and other news and then I got up and told everyone what was happening to Maureen. They learned to make the announcements at the end and let the prayer requests have a separate place.

Reverend Sayer made more visits to the hospital and to our house. He learned about Dingmans Bridge from traveling to visit Maureen at Newton Hospital. The first time he ever crossed the bridge was to visit her. Early on I left the room when he came, but as the days wore on, Maureen told me to stay. She didn't want me far from her. Besides, Maureen was reserved. I guess you could call it a blue-collar dignity. And she couldn't have long talks with Reverend Sayer anymore because she got so tired. After a little conversation Maureen's breathing became strained and talking was an effort.

But Steve knew when his presence was helpful and when it was a burden. After they talked for 10 or 15 minutes, he would ask, "Maureen, is this getting to be too much?" Maureen was straightforward and said, "I just can't today," if Steve called and asked about a visit.

During one of these visits, Maureen and he sat together to pick hymns for her funeral. She wanted to take the burden from him and me and take responsibility for herself. She faced everything head on, and the planning kept Maureen going. She wanted to leave as much of herself as she could.

Transfusion needed
Medical Record 04/10/98
Office Records
'Spoke with nurse from Cancer Unit in PA, patient complaining of dizziness, fatigue, bruising and petechiae. She is concerned she will need a transfusion. Stat CBC ordered.

By now I was familiar with the terms the doctors and other medical people used. I learned to stop them each time and ask them to explain, to tell me so I could know what Maureen's body was doing and what they were doing to her. I learned more than anyone should ever know, but I never stopped asking. Maureen was still not making enough blood cells or platelets. She was like a beautiful car running on very thin gasoline, doing her best to keep going, but getting slower and slower. The dizziness and the bruising were all part of it. Small spots erupted on her skin called Petechia that came from the small blood vessels bursting underneath the surface.

Platelet transfusions
Medical Record 04/14/98
Newton Memorial Hospital
Platelet transfusion for thrombocytopenia.

Medical Record 04/20/98
Office Visit
'She is still bleeding. Neumega was ordered. she will be having a transfusion for platelets tonight.'

Medical Record 04/20/98
Newton Memorial Hospital
Platelet transfusion for thrombocytopenia

The battle for platelets became primary. Maureen couldn't do it for herself and she never would again. The cancer was too strong and the chemotherapy and radiation had literally burned her out. The Neumega was supposed to help increase Maureen's production of platelets, but we were still injecting it and those shots were murder on Maureen. She screamed every time they were given to her. Like every other drug, the doctors told me what to watch for. They told me to get her back to the hospital if her breath became very short, if she had chest pains or was light headed. If Maureen had previous problems with her lungs, Neumega could make things worse. So far, her lungs were O.K., but she broke out in hives.

After more transfusions, the platelets stabilized a little, so the doctors went after the cancer again. This time it was Navelbine or 'Vinorelbine' which we injected into Maureen in a nearly clear yellow fluid. The problem with this chemotherapy, just like all the others is that it slows blood cell production in the bone marrow. It was a nightmare merry-go-round. Maureen needed blood cells, but she needed to fight the cancer. She was in a corner. I could hardly pay attention to the tiredness and light headedness they warned me about this time. Maureen was nothing but tired already. I did watch her for fevers. Any kind of infection would wipe her out in a hurry.

New chemotherapy
Medical Record 04/23/98
Office Visit
'Since having platelet transfusions on several occasions over the past several weeks she is no longer bleeding from the nose and from the rectum.
We have decided to go with Navelbine as the next chemo considering everything else that she has already had.'

At this point the doctors told the lawyers to get the last deposition from Maureen. They didn't know how long she would last. On April 25th, I brought Maureen to the lawyers' office for the third deposition. Maureen sat with oxygen tubes in her nose and took sips of water every few minutes. She could barely speak because her lungs were full of fluid. She was fabulous. She knew the law suit wasn't going to help her at all, and she made me promise to give some of the money from the lawsuit to the church. She was determined to see it through to the end. And she did. She did everything she needed to do. She was still angry and she wanted justice for Erik and Ryan. Maureen sat in the lawyers' office and let them make their tape.

She wore a wig that looked identical to her own hair, identical to how she Looked when she first walked into the office in Stroudsburg. It was eerie because they did her initial interview in that conference room and again for the final interview. That morning, same as before, she put on an outfit and made up her face so no one could tell that her body was betraying her. She answered some of the same questions again and the defense lawyers wanted to know why she thought an ultrasound was better than a mammogram. Maureen never showed her anger. She answered them each time like it was a question about which dish detergent she liked better. When we were in the car, she closed her eyes and let herself slump. I don't know what was holding her upright during the deposition.

Only a few days later, Maureen was struggling to breath. This deposition took place soon after she began taking the Navelbine, which made it hard for her to breathe sometimes. Her breath had been short for a while, but now it was serious. I called the doctor and he told me to get to the hospital fast.

Platelet transfusion; cell biopsy
Medical Record 4/27/98
Newton Memorial Hospital
Admitted with a diagnosis of Bilateral Pleural Effusion &
Thrombocytopenia
Chief complaint was shortness of breath.
Transfusion of platelets due to markedly decreased platelet
count of 9,000.
Left paracentesis performed -133 cc obtained and sent for
cytology-results were malignant with cells consistent with
metastatic ductal carcinoma.

Medical Record 4/28/98
Newton Memorial Hospital
Discharged.

Maureen's lungs were full of fluid from the cancer. They had to do an emergency lung tap where they drew out the fluid and sent it to the lab. Newton Hospital was now monitoring her cancer around the clock. I was right there. I watched the cancer coming out of her through a tube and into a little dish. I measured the cc's and wrote it down. I knew more about Maureen's cancer than the oncologist and he'd be the first to admit it. I knew more about Maureen's stem cell than anyone at Newton Hospital and they would admit it. I'm not asking for a pat on the back and I'm not bragging. I just had to know.

Lesions; Neumega injections
Medical Record 4/30/98
Office Visit
Macular skin lesions noted.
Prescription for Famvir
Husband taught to give Neumega injections for decreased platelet count.

At the beginning of May I learned to inject Maureen with Neumega, which was in its clinical trials in Hackensack. The nurses at Newton Hospital hadn't even seen Neumega yet. They were a wonderful support team. I had prescriptions from Hackensack that I mixed, and these were drugs that the Newton Memorial nurses had never seen. That's the way it was, because Maureen had lung cancer too. As soon as less than 50 cc of fluid came out of her lungs in a six-hour period, we could go home. The procedure seemed to work pretty well at the hospital, but I found out later that there was so much cancer, it had clogged the tubes, deceiving us as to how much fluid was coming out. We went home and Maureen's breathing came a little easier.

Maureen was always asleep or in pain, but she knew what I was going through. It was the 3rd of May. It was morning and I asked her if she wanted to do anything. There were always things that she wanted to take care of, and she had written them down, like the names of all the funeral homes. Maureen wanted to visit funeral homes. I said, "O.K., let's go." The name of one I liked was on her list, so I said, "Let's go there first."

Maureen could walk a little, so as soon as I got her in the car, she said, "I want to stop at the store first." She said the name of the local department store.

I pulled into the parking lot and came around to her door to help her get out. When I opened the door, she said, "Bill, I can't walk."

"What do you mean you can't walk? Your legs won't move?"

"No, I can't breathe."

"I'm taking you to the hospital." I started to close the door.

"No," she said, "Can you go get me a wheelchair?"

Going into the store and getting a wheelchair for Maureen just killed me. She walked everywhere before that and she loved to shop. I never thought it was going to come down to a wheelchair. I went into the store and got her a wheelchair and came out and put her in it.

"What do you want at the store?"

We had talked a few days before about buying things for the boys for their eighteenth and twenty-first birthdays and for graduations. Maureen wanted to be a part of everything. She didn't want to be left out, and she was planning ahead.

When we got inside the store, Maureen said, "Take me to the jewelry counter."

The clerk saw us and asked what we wanted. Maureen pointed to the men's wedding bands. My wedding ring had broken years ago when I was doing a landscaping job, and I never replaced it. Maureen picked out a simple gold band, not too thick for $79 and put it on my hand right there in the store. I don't remember paying for it. I just remember kneeling next to her in the wheelchair and watching her fingers slide the ring into place. Everything around me disappeared. I saw her hands and mine.

We left the store and Maureen said, "Let's go to the funeral home," as if we were going to pick out new kitchen chairs. Her breathing was getting worse, so I told her again I wanted to take her to the hospital,

"No."

"Come on, Maureen. You need to go to the hospital." We were back in the car by this time.

"I'm not going anywhere but the funeral parlor. If you won't drive me I'll call a taxi." She was looking straight out the windshield.

"Maureen, you don't have to do this." I couldn't take my eyes off her. I was afraid she was going to lose her breath for good right there.

"Just drive, Bill.

It was about the worst argument we ever had and she wasn't giving in.

The funeral home was a three-story building with displays on each floor. I helped Maureen from the car to inside the front door. As soon as the door shut, Maureen sat right down on the stairs inside the building. She could barely talk. She was having a real hard time, and she was cold. I covered her with one of the blankets I always carried, and she sat at the base of the stairs trying to catch her breath.

The funeral director came out and was real polite as Maureen told him what she wanted. First she wanted to look at the memorial cards then she wanted to look at flowers, but she didn't have the strength to get up and go into the different rooms to look at them. The funeral director and I brought her samples while she sat on the step. She nodded and said, "That's pretty," until she found what she wanted. When she looked at the pictures of flower arrangements, I sat down next to her and turned the pages. I couldn't talk. Maureen knew I was upset, because she loved flowers so much.

"You're not going to cry at my funeral, Bill," she said stubborn, but kind of teasing. "You're not."

I put my arm around her and she put her head on my shoulder, her breath coming hard. "If I'm going to be the center of attention, I want a party." She pointed to the bouquet she wanted.

I heard her words, but I was listening to the air squeezing in and out of her chest. Next it was the caskets and the urns; they were on the second and third floor, and the elevator was broken. I put my arms around Maureen to carry her, but I couldn't. She was so swollen from all the fluids and she weighed over 170 pounds. I was sick and weak from not sleeping, not eating, taking care of Maureen. I had lost 40 pounds. I wanted to carry her up those steps, but I didn't have the strength.

Maureen did three steps at a time. She went up three steps and sat down. We waited until she caught her breath. The funeral director was a wonderful gentleman; he went every step with us. We got to the second floor and Maureen looked over every casket model, until she was standing next to one she liked.

"Do you think I'll look good in this?" she asked me.

"No," I said. I couldn't help it. How could I say she would look good in a casket? I saw shadows moving in her eyes, and I said, "You'll look better than good. You'll be gorgeous."

It took an hour from the time we arrived at the funeral home to the time she picked out a casket. "Where are the urns?" she asked. The urns were on the third floor. The funeral director offered to bring every urn down to her, but Maureen wanted to go up and see them on her own. She made it. She picked out a teal ceramic urn. And then she made it down. When we got home, Maureen picked out the clothes for her funeral and the make up she wanted put on her face. Then I took her to the hospital.

Lung infection/Chest tube inserted/Platelet transfusion
Medical Record 5/03/98
Newton Memorial Hospital
Admitted via the Emergency Room with difficulty breathing.
Diagnosis: recurrent malignant Pleural Infection
Chest tube inserted due to persistent metastatic pleural effusion.
Several platelet transfusions during this hospitalization.
Chemical pleurodesis attempted without success for pleural effusion.
Condition deteriorated during this admission.

Maureen went back to the hospital for lung tap to her right lung. This time it was much deeper, much more violent. It was a terrible thing to witness. She spent the next eleven days in the hospital getting worse and worse. I stayed with her almost around the clock. The boys came in to visit, and I taught them how to manage the pump on the morphine drip. They wanted to help so the doctor and I didn't have to do it.

Patty came in to visit Maureen in Newton Hospital that week. Maureen and she had a great talk. But Maureen's mom and sister visited too and that was difficult for all of them. They were scared and sad, and I know they felt helpless looking at Maureen.

Mother's Day came and I remembered that Maureen always wanted a little electric keyboard. I was holding her hand and Erik and Ryan were taking turns pumping the morphine button, when I remembered. The morphine finally gave her some peace and she fell asleep, so we snuck out of the hospital and drove fast to the store. We told the nurses we were leaving, and we bought a keyboard and brought it back. Maureen couldn't form whole sentences by this time. She was so full of drugs and the cancer was wiping her out. Her mouth was a mess of sores. We used medical swabs to clean it, but she couldn't chew.

After a half hour or so, she woke up and saw the boys. She lit up like a star, she was that happy to see them. When she saw the keyboard, it was like the sun coming out after a terrible storm. She smiled so big and she played LeAnn Rime's *Looking Through Your Eyes*, every word, and sang it clear as anything.

Honest to God, the nurses, everyone, stopped and looked at her, it was like a light came on and a star bloomed. They all stood to listen to Maureen sing. That was Sunday, Mother's Day.

Maureen wanted to go home and die in the sun room. On Thursday, May 14th, I said I was taking her home, but the hospital didn't want to release her. They said she wouldn't live through the night.

"No," I told them. "That's not going to work. I can get her home in an hour. She doesn't ask for much. She wants to die at home in the sun room."

I rode with her in the back of an ambulance. An EMT rode in back with us while another drove. I held Maureen the whole way, talking to her, telling her about the sun room and how it was waiting just for her. We were halfway home when Maureen stopped breathing. The EMT got air going in and out of her again, but a few miles later, her breath stopped again. "Hold on, Maureen. Come on, don't give up!" I grabbed her arm and shook her. I yelled at her too. "You don't want to die here. Everything's set up at home. Don't die now." I meant it. The ambulance drivers knew I meant it too. I yelled at them, "Get her home!" The driver stepped on the gas, and the EMT and I held onto Maureen. We pulled into the driveway and she was still breathing. The EMT's face was white. Maybe he thought I was crazy.

Hospice
Medical Record 5/14/98
Newton Memorial Hospital
Discharged to Hospice Care in Home

Medical Record 5/14/98
Admitted to Hospice
Nurses to come to home 3x week
Bill Thiel is primary care giver at this point
Oxygen @ 4 liters continuous
Admission Hospice notes: described Maureen as alert and disoriented with visual and auditory hallucinations and described Maureen as fearful of hallucinations.

Maureen's friend, Cheryl from Florida, came on Thursday, and stayed with us. She arrived just in time at Newark Airport to get to Newton Hospital and drive behind the ambulance. Hospice met us at our house. The hospice people and the EMTs got the bed and the oxygen tank in. I had Maureen's bed set up in the sunroom. Maureen never, ever asked for anything. She always asked, "What can I give?" That was her huge heart. I gave her the sunroom and a little wrought iron shelf to make it pretty for her.

She made it home on Thursday and the pain management began. By that time I couldn't give her the Neumega shots for platelets. She begged me, "Please don't give me the shots." They hurt her so bad. From then on nights at the house were a nightmare. Every night, Maureen moaned and screamed. Nothing we did softened her pain. The screaming was unbearable. The boys tried to sleep at the house, but it was too hard for them to hear their mom in pain. They stayed together at a neighbor's house every night and then split up during the day to go to friends' houses. I don't remember where they were all those days. I owe those good people for their generosity and understanding. It wasn't easy on any of us. When Maureen was in the hospital, just like months before, I took the boys for rides to talk and explain. Erik realized during one of those rides that his mom wasn't going to make it.

On Friday, May 15th, Patty and three other women from the neighborhood came to visit. Maureen didn't know who they were. She cried out, she was in so much pain. Later that day, Helen Sheffo, came over. She had made two quilts with six squares on each. One square had a fabric a pair of scissors, because Maureen was a beautician; another had a campfire, because Helen and her husband were our camping buddies. A third square had a Christmas tree, to remember the year we sold Christmas trees on the side of the road. Maureen loved angels, so there are angels sewed on a fourth square. The fifth square had cloth figures of two small boys, Erik and Ryan. And there was a blank square.

Both quilts were exactly the same, each with one blank square. I had no idea what she was going to do. She hadn't stopped crying since she came in the door, but she took out hand paint and painted Maureen's hand. She pressed Maureen's hand on each quilt. Helen gave one quilt to Erik and one to Ryan. That was her good-bye and her thank you to Maureen. Maureen touched many women's hearts in that community and church.

By that time, though, Maureen didn't know who anybody was. Maureen said only one thing now. "I wuv ya Biw, I wuv ya Biw, I wuv ya Biw." "I love you, Bill." There were no more sentences. She mumbled that over and over when she wasn't screaming in pain. I hung sheets around Maureen's bed to keep the air still around her, but even a small breeze would move the sheets and send her screaming again. I couldn't touch her. I couldn't hug her.

Severe pain; hallucinations
Medical Record 5/15/98
Telephone call to doctor from Hospice Nurse
'Patient in severe pain. Unable to continue with current treatment.'
Order for Duragesic patch given nurse.
Hospice notes: lethargic, restless with auditory and visual hallucinations patient cries out with pain in various areas of the body.
Foley catheter in place for urinary output.

Maureen was done. There weren't going to be any more surgeries, treatments or transfusions. There would be no more shots. She just screamed. Erik and Ryan came in to see her and left. It was too hard for them. It was never too hard for me; I could always be around her.

On Saturday morning, May 16th, Cheryl and I were taking care of Maureen. We sat with her and talked to her. Cheryl sang church songs. I listened for a while, then I stood and told Cheryl I was going outside for a little air. I got up to leave and Cheryl said, "Don't go."

I sat back down just as close to Maureen as I could without hurting her and told her what a blessing she was. I told her she was going to fit right in with the angels. I knew it was time, because she wouldn't take her eyes off me. I told her I'd be there as soon as the Lord was done with me here, and we could start up right where we left off. Right before the lump and the scream took our life together away. I bent my head real close and I told her what I had told her fifteen years before.

"Maureen, you are my wife and you have made me whole. When we are in heaven, we aren't going to have to change the way we make love. I already know you're a piece of heaven."

Maureen let out a sigh and let all her screaming go. She let go of all the pain and all the fear. She let go of the cancer. She let go of her life.

I closed her eyes and I closed her mouth. I had to do it twice to make them stay closed. I didn't cry. I was dying inside, but I had no tears.

Last record
Medical Record 5/16/98
Expired.

Maureen died a terrible death. It wasn't fair. When she died and her physical heart was gone, half of me was ripped away, leaving an empty hole. I went on with half a heart. Fifteen years with Maureen wasn't long enough. I loved Maureen more than anyone will ever know, and I thank God for the time I had with her. Some people will live a lifetime and never know a love like we had.

After Maureen died and I had called the funeral parlor, I went to the lake to find Ryan. We walked out to the end of the dock. "Ryan," I said, "Mom's gone. She died just a little while ago at the house."

He looked out over the lake then he squinted up at me. "Is she out of pain, Dad?"

I nodded. Ryan nodded too and then he smiled at me. "I just don't want her to hurt any more."

"I know," I said. "It's O.K. to be happy that the pain is over."

Erik was down at the lake too, but by the time we found him, Maureen's sister Katheryn had told him. When I saw him his face said, "No that couldn't happen." So I told him all over again. I told him his Mom was peaceful now and the pain would never reach her again. I think Erik had frozen up inside little by little over the past year and this day was the final layer of ice. He looked at me, but he was inside a glass wall. The boys told their friends they had to go home and from there, the news spread through the neighborhood.

The funeral was beautiful and awful. It was one of the largest services our community had ever had, and the funeral director said he had never seen anything like it. Nearly all of our church congregation was there and most of our neighbors from the Pocono Mountain Lake Estates. The whole company I worked for, Steve Willands, shut down that day so that everyone could attend. Even the lawyers, Michael MacDonald and Malcolm McGregor as well as Marcia Kohanski came.

The funeral home was filled with the flowers and people Maureen loved. Over 350 people packed into the rooms and stood along the sides. She was right there at the heart of it in her silver casket. The light came in bright and soft through the windows, and I know she was happy resting right there. The Reverend Sayer spoke to us about how tragic and even wasteful it felt, but that Maureen had shown us how to meet our worst challenges with courage and dignity. He said that he too felt like her life was incomplete and that it was our job to honor her by completing her life for her. He said we could do that by remembering her generous and giving heart and following her example. We sang all the hymns Maureen had picked out and then we played "Stairway to Heaven" by Led Zeppelin as we carried her out to the hearse.

People gave me their condolences and I could see in their eyes that they were stunned. I could see myself in their faces. None of us had been ready. I thought I would be prepared after all we'd been through, but I wasn't. Everyone looked so shocked and concerned for the boys and me.

At the cemetery, people stood in small clumps, dabbing at their eyes. I remember a man standing by himself next to a tree and sobbing. The boys were lost among the grown ups. They shook hands with people and watched everyone's face to get some kind of answers, but none of us had anything that could help. I didn't cry at the funeral. It was like a movie Maureen had written and everything went as planned. It wasn't real. But when she was cremated, I fell apart. I knew the exact time. It didn't seem right and I couldn't stand it. I knew how much Maureen loved her teal urn, but the idea of my beautiful girl turned to ash tore me up.

We buried her beside her polished granite heart, and it would have been all right with me if they had buried me right then too. A heart-shaped juniper shrub stands in front of the headstone. I planted pampas grass on either side of and a dog wood tree stands behind it. A dwarf lilac shrub grows to the side. Erik, Ryan and I put a wooden love-seat with wrought iron sides beside the grave. We painted the slats red, white and blue. Half of Maureen's ashes are buried there in the teal ceramic urn. The rest the boys and I keep until we can let them go out at sea.

Patty Flotz came to check on us a few weeks after Maureen died and to tell me that she and some of Maureen's friends were at the lake that day. It was spring, a blue sky, calm day. They were picnicking, she said, picnicking and things were kind of quiet. All of a sudden, out of nowhere, a wind blew through. Patty said it lasted for a just few seconds, swaying the trees, and putting everything in motion, a real strong wind. She said it was a little scary. Then she told me all the women looked at one another and said, "That was Maureen."

I wasn't surprised.

Chapter Six

The Verdict

For two weeks after Maureen died, I couldn't leave the house. I made sure the boys had food and the neighbors watched out for them. I sat on our bed and stared at Maureen's clothes in the closet. Maybe one of the boys came in and said something, or maybe I realized Maureen would have told me to get up, but I finally made some dinner and started thinking about what to do. I tried to follow all the things Maureen had asked of me. She had said, "Make sure if I die that all my things go to the Bushkill Outreach," an organization that distributes food and clothes to low-income families She had a lot of clothes, so I took everything out of the closet. I folded her dresses and her pants into neat piles like a robot. Then I went to her bureau. Everything was already folded: stacks of t-shirts with pansies or cardinals on the front, or striped button-down-the-front shirts. They smelled like Maureen, clean and ready to go. My hands got unsteady and a pile slid. I got angry and grabbed a bunch to put back on top of the bureau, but instead of just shirts I felt something hard. I folded back the cloth and saw a cassette tape. I didn't stop to think why it was there; I went into the kitchen and put it in the cassette player. The voice that came out of that box froze me.

> It's Thursday, the 11th, 1997. Yesterday I had my stem cells removed, so now I'm just sitting here waiting to go to the hospital next week and have the high dose chemo.
>
> Hah! I've got to admit something. I'm scared to death. I'm very, very scared.
>
> I guess the reason that I'm doing this tape is I want you three guys to know that I love you all very, very much. I really do. And I keep asking why me. You must know I ask "why me?" all the time. You probably ask "why you?" I hate the fact

that I have cancer. I hate it. I try to figure out all the time. What did I do in my life? If I had to get it, then please let it respond to chemo, but damn it, it's not responding. I just pray to God. You don't know how I pray that it responds to this stem cell, that the stem cell therapy kills it. It has to catch it, not to kill me. You know I do a lot of sleeping these days. I think it's a combination of I'm weak and when I sleep my mind doesn't work. So I just sleep the days and nights away without thinking about what's happening. If I don't make it through this stem cell chemotherapy, I want you to know that the last fourteen years have been the best years of my life. It seems like yesterday I lived in MGTP and met your father. Seems like at that time I was real down and out too. I didn't think I'd ever find anybody who would appreciate me for who I was. Until I met Dad. And he's never failed me in fourteen years. He showed me a love that I had never known. I hope, Erik and Ryan that you will each meet a girl and fall in love just like me and Daddy fell in love. It's not easy to find, but if you take your time you'll find it. I know you will.

Erik, be good in your life. I know you and Ryan squabble and fight and bicker with one another, but I know you love him. Take care of each other. Be each other's friend. Stay close to each other. Keep the family together, so that your kids will have cousins to play with and at Christmas you'll get together.

I don't like the fact that this is taking us so close to Christmas, but I pray, I just pray and pray and pray I get to see the new year, I get to see 1998. And if I can get to see 1998, I know things will be better. Just these last few months of 1997 have been real tough on me.

And Ryan, know that I love you. I'll always love all of you, always. Even though I might not be here with you, I'll still love all of you. Take care of yourself Ryan. This is so unfair. Everything about this disease is so unfair. But what can I do?

Wait, I've got to blow my nose, guys.

I want you to be good boys all your life. Take care of your father. And do those things for one another. I hope to see you this weekend. I hope you come to Pennsylvania this weekend and I'm going to give you guys the biggest hugs I've ever given you. I had fun with you this past weekend at Dan's house. I hope your arm's all right Ryan. That's what I warned John about. Watch what you're doing and don't hurt yourselves. It doesn't take much to really break an arm or injure yourself. You both have to take care of yourself.

And Erik, those trick things that you do on bikes, I don't know, sometimes I wish you wouldn't do all those things, 'cause I'm afraid for you. Don't be so daring, it's not worth it. Life does have consequences. Eat right, make good friends, stay away from drugs. Please don't smoke and be loving and helpful and caring people.

That's all I can think of to say right now. I love you.

I stood there in a trance. Hearing Maureen's voice was a miracle and a torture. I heard the boys coming, so I pulled the tape out and put it in my pocket. They weren't ready for it, so I had to hold everything in. With that tape in my head, I started doing some wash, cleaning the bathroom and getting the boys off to school a little better than before.

Hospice had come and taken the bed out of the sunroom. I hadn't touched anything since then. After taking the clothes to Bushkill Outreach, I went into the sunroom and started pushing things around, trying to put things into some kind of normal order. Nothing made sense, and I didn't care. I pushed a chair from one side of the room to the other and it caught on the rug in the middle of the floor, rumpling it into folds and pulling it sideways. There was Maureen on the floor outlined in paint. She must have lain on the floor and traced herself while the boys and I were out, before she got too sick to move around by herself. Next to it she wrote, "I am here for you." It was just a simple outline, and the hands were open. I knelt down and put my hands on hers, put my whole body against her drawing. It hurt so bad I could hardly breathe. I knew she put the drawing there for the boys, but I had to put the rug over it, so I didn't see it every time I walked by.

And that wasn't the end of it. When I unpacked the summer clothes for the boys, there were notes from Maureen telling us if we found the note, that meant she wasn't there to help, but how much she loves us and not to worry, she will be watching over us. I didn't find the notes in the Christmas ornaments until the second year after she died. It said, "Merry Christmas, Bill, Erik and Ryan. When you put the star at the top, that's me smiling down on you." Most of the time I hoped she wasn't watching.

The first four months were nothing but hell for Erik and Ryan and me. All we did was argue and fight. The nucleus of our home was gone and we were nothing but three atoms running around with no home base. We fought, we argued. Ryan was 10, Erik was 12. The boys came home from school and made a bigger mess of the house. I wasn't the best cleaning person. Ryan's teacher said he came to school and just sat. The house was boring and empty. I thought a dog might help. We called her Runt because she was so little, but she only made the mess worse. The boys fought horribly. Erik would kick Ryan in the back, and I didn't pay attention to what they fought about. Ryan never had his friends over anymore, but Erik's friends still came by, so Ryan started hanging around with the older boys.

I tried to go back to work. Steven Willand, my boss, knew that I was going to be out of work a long time. The company kept me on the payroll even when I wasn't working to keep my medical insurance going. I felt so guilty, so I stopped them from paying me. When I did go back to work, I didn't want any money from them. I had a little bit of money from the life insurance policy, enough for a couple of months, so I worked without pay for Steven Willand to pay back all the money.

It helped me to be back at work, but there were problems at home. The boys had to get themselves off to school. They missed the bus, fought with each other and missed a lot of school. I got phone calls all the time with those two screaming at each other. Erik never talked about how much Maureen's death hurt him. When he was with friends, he watched their moms and his face would shut down. It bothered him so much that he quit going places with his friends. It was too hard for him to see the other moms pick up their kids or doing things with them. It drove him crazy, but he never said a word. He started smoking cigarettes and drinking about that time and Ryan followed his example. I didn't want to be at home because we were all so angry. I was running away. I was losing it. I couldn't figure out a way to heal. Every once in while we'd have a good day like when I took them to Dorny Park. They had fun, but I couldn't handle seeing all the couples together.

At work I saw pain in everyone's eyes for Maureen and for me. I went to church and it was worse. Every time they saw me, they saw Maureen, and I knew it. I couldn't go to church anymore. There was sorrow everywhere I looked, and everywhere reminders of how Maureen was loved. I couldn't think about healing. The two of us were woven together, how could I let that go?

I didn't make the best choices after Maureen died. People wanted to help and they wanted me to let them in. Many people in the church cared for us and wanted to help the boys. They offered support that would have been helpful. Everyone was shocked and wanted to share our grief. I couldn't face any of it, and I didn't know what to do, so I faded away from the community.

I was drifting, trying to find something not connected to Maureen. I tried to let go of it all. I met a woman named Jenny four months after Maureen died, and

I moved to Wilkes-Barre the following April in 1999. People were surprised and bewildered when I moved my family away. The community had no place to put their feelings for Maureen.

Jenny tried to fill the void for all three of us, but it was all wrong. It wasn't Jenny's fault, it was mine. Ryan adapted better than Erik or I. He thought the move was exciting, so I moved him in with Jenny before Erik and me, to keep the boys from fighting. The school was O.K., and Ryan fit in quickly.

I thought it would be a new start, with new schools for the boys. But it got worse for Erik and Ryan. I tried to run away from Maureen, but there was no running away from anything. It didn't work at all for Jenny and me, so it went back to being Erik, Ryan and me. I took a job with Federal Express, bought my own delivery van, a franchise deal, and worked long hours. I was self-employed, and able to manage only the bare necessities. I was in denial. I knew I had to be strong for the boys, but I never took the time to stop and let everything that had happened sink in. I worked as hard as I could, but I didn't pay enough attention to what the boys really needed. I didn't want to get up in the morning, but I had to and take care of the boys. This was something I had never done before. It had been Maureen's job. I did what she had always told me to do, and that was go to work. The bottom had fallen out of our world.

I was a very unlovable person during that period. I was irrational, and doing a lot of the 'poor pitiful me' thing. Maureen never did that. It was very wrong on my part, but I had just gone through a life-altering experience that I didn't know how to handle. Everywhere I went was misery, especially at night.

These were the long years of terrible dreams. I didn't know what to do, so I called Malcolm MacGregor, the lawyer. He told me to call a psychiatrist, and I tried several. I worked on it on my own and with their help. I tried to concentrate and think about the good times with Maureen, but the therapists knew it was going to take time because of what I had gone through and how close I was to Maureen.

In the dreams Maureen was alive, but she had cancer, no hair and we knew she was going to die. I lived it all over again, always with Maureen bald and mad; dreams of her fighting because she wanted to help other women. Then it got worse. In the dreams Maureen had been buried, but I had to go back to the funeral home and say, "We have to bury her again, could you give me a discount?" I argued with the funeral director over and over. That dream put me into cold sweats.

During this time I went on line to LOVE@oal and talked to women over the Internet. I met over 50 women that way. I met them at a safe public place, hoping destiny or the chemistry would be right. I was so lonely, with half my heart gone. It was too much to ask someone to fill that void. I hoped, but if I was doing something in my dream with somebody else, Maureen showed up too.

One dream stands out from all the rest. I was sitting at my kitchen table having coffee, when a huge, hazy white light came into the room. It was Maureen, glowing. I thought, "Here's my angel". I wasn't upset or worried. I said, "Hi, Maureen, would you like a cup of coffee?" She said calmly, "No, I'm only going to be here for a moment. I want you to pursue the boys' dream. Their skate dream." She vanished and I woke up sweating. Erik and Ryan wanted to own a skate park, a roller-blade and skate board park. They had been practicing and were really good. We built a small "park" in our back yard with ramps, tubes and rails. The weird thing was that they started doing those things after Maureen died.

From that day on, I tried to love the boys for the two of us. It had seemed an easy promise to make, but it was a hard one to keep. Every time I looked at them, I saw Maureen, but she couldn't see them do anything unless she was up there watching.

All through this time, I tried to tell Maureen's story to save lives. I talked to women about early breast cancer detection and how doctors sometime fail to diagnose and treat breast lumps. I was on the phone and on the Internet with every cancer organization I could think of. Maureen asked me to do this, and I was not going to let her down.

In 2002, I met Lisa Neary, and we started dating. Pretty soon I realized how much I liked her. I was trying to fall in love just as I had promised Maureen, but nothing was easy. I tried to tell Maureen about Lisa in my dreams, but I always woke up just at the moment of saying Lisa's name. One night I stayed asleep long enough to tell Maureen about Lisa. Maureen said, "I know." Is that closure? It was the last dream I had about Maureen.

In the background of everything was the lawsuit. It was up to me to keep it going for the boys. The lawsuit had Maureen's name on it, not mine, and her signature was on all the legal papers. I met with the lawyers for six years after Maureen died, and they gathered information, witnesses and evidence. Maureen's depositions were done, so the lawyers put together a team to prove the first three doctors were wrong in their diagnosis.

Most people have an image of what lawyers are like. They take people to court, sue them and they're done. It's all business and each case is a way for the firm to make money. That's true most of the time, but not for these lawyers. Maureen had a story to tell and they knew it. By the spring of 2004, I was talking to Malcolm and Michael nearly every day. Even then, even though I knew this was what Maureen wanted, I had a hard time seeing the point. One day, I point blank asked Malcolm why he and the firm took the case.

"Maureen was very focused right from the outset," Malcolm told me. She knew what she wanted to do. She was angry, but that didn't get in the way of what she knew was right. She condensed her story quickly: 'Look, I first went to this doctor in November of 1994, and I put his hand on my breast, I showed him where it was. I showed each doctor every time after that. They always told me it was O.K. Nobody told me to worry. The fourth doctor diagnosed me with cancer.' Maureen knew the magnitude of her story with 47 out of 47 nodes cancerous. She knew it was bad news when she came to talk to us."

Malcolm and Michael explained everything to me as they went along. They said there had been a breach in the standard of care. The doctors did not do the tests they needed to do. A biopsy could have diagnosed the cancer earlier. Right from the beginning, all those legal factors were there. Malcolm said, "We could smell those as soon as she started talking. Right from the start, Maureen was a very compelling, powerful personality, as a witness. We knew she would be quite good. What was outrageous and made the case particularly attractive, was that she gave the doctors everything they needed to do the right thing."

Maureen literally put the doctors' hands on the lump in her breast and said, "Here it is." She directed them to it. They didn't have to look for it or wonder where it was. Malcolm and Michael were also impressed that Maureen did more than the doctors asked her to. If Maureen was told to have a mammogram in a year, she came back in six months. Maureen played by the rules and she lost, because the doctors let her down. Maureen wanted to do something so no other woman would have to go through this.

I began to understand that what had happened to Maureen was outrageous, and from the beginning the lawyers knew it was a huge case. As the case proceeded, it was long, hard slogging, unexciting work. There were days when Malcolm told me he wondered if he was ever going to synthesize all the details into the simple powerful story that he knew it was."

As they prepared for the trial, Malcolm, Michael and Marcia developed a friendship with the boys. When I first brought Erik and Ryan back to the lawyers, they didn't want to talk at all. I told them, "You have to talk to these guys; it's for your mother's case." It took them a while, but after listening to all the pieces they got it, and they were great. They were true and honest through the whole process.

I watched Malcolm ask the boys questions. Erik especially hated talking about his mom. His face was a storm of anger. After, when the boys were in another room, I told Malcolm this was too hard for them.

"I know," he said. "This is probably going to be the most intense time of your life. I don't want to scare you.

"Can't we just settle?"

"We'd love to, but we have to go to trial. Maureen wanted to see this through, and it bothered her that she wasn't going to be here. I don't think she cared about the outcome; she just wanted to tell her own story. That's why it's so important to do this the right way."

The lawyers talked to our friends from the Pocono Mountain Lake Estates and from the church. They wanted people to let the jury know what they had lost when Maureen died. It was hard enough for them to lose her, but to go into court and re-open that wound was an awful thing to face. I understood. Most agreed to testify because the trial had a purpose.

Some people were upset with me because I was with Lisa. Maureen held our family together and after she died, I fell apart. I hit rock-bottom and I made some bad decisions, but Lisa isn't one of them. I never should have sold the house or uprooted the kids. Maybe some of our friends are still angry at me for that.

Some people did not agree with the trial on principle. Maureen hadn't discussed the trial or her reasons behind it with many people, so a few might believe I wasn't putting her illness to rest. Many people view lawsuits as wrong, as mean, and a way to get money. All the money in the world wouldn't bring Maureen back. It wasn't an issue of anyone saying bad things or getting rich.

When the testimonies came, they came easily. It was a pleasure for them to talk about Maureen, that's the kind of person that she was. They didn't have to think deeply about why they liked her. Everyone was very forthcoming, and the lawyers had to whittle the witness list down. Neighbor after neighbor came forward, people who hadn't seen her for years because she had been sick came forward. Revered Steve Sayer came forward. All these good people came to testify on Maureen's behalf. No one had to coax testimony out of them. All Malcolm or Michael or Marcia had to say was, "Maureen Thiel," and they started talking. She was like the thumping heart beat of this little community and the thumping heartbeat of her family.

Before the trial, Malcolm and Michael tested the case before a mock jury chosen randomly from voter registration lists. This group met at East Stroudsburg University three weeks before trial to hear a summary of the case and see exhibits. The lawyers made many presentations to them, focusing on the worst problems and difficulties of the case. One difficulty was how to present Doctor Berger to the jury. Doctor Berger was a woman that Maureen trusted. Malcolm and Michael were concerned that the jury would sympathize with the doctor. But Doctor Berger's personality spoke for the lawyers. When her part of the case was put before the mock jury, the members, especially the women, became angry. Their response to Doctor Berger was clear: "Here is one woman coming to another woman for help, and the doctor let her down. Maureen Thiel specifically chose a woman doctor believing she would listen better and be more aware."

Malcolm and Michael also worried that a jury might get confused and argue about the exact location of the breast lump. The medical records placed it at five or six o'clock. The test jury saw the chart and a picture of Maureen's breast and evaluated where the lumps were found. The mock jury proved that no one was going to argue over such a small difference, and they had no difficulty agreeing that there was a delay of two years and four months in her diagnosis.

From the mock jury's response, the legal team developed a clear exhibit. It was a flip chart that started in 1999 with a clean bill of health. In sequence the chart showed all of the doctor's visits, mammograms, ultrasounds, and final diagnosis. The final statement read, "521 days with no aspirations, no biopsy: a two-year, four-month delay." The lawyers anticipated problems and road tested everything.

Malcolm and Michael reviewed the case file repeatedly, turning old information into new strategies. They looked at the testimonies from different angles. Malcolm went to the American Trial Lawyers' Association Program at Harvard in Cambridge, MA, a 'trial lawyer's boot camp', very sophisticated, very intense. He brought this case to test the opening and the closing. He was worried. The lawyers at Harvard gave him honest reactions and told him the case was powerful. They told Malcolm to focus on Maureen and stay there, because it was a very simple, powerful story. Malcolm and Michael told me they were very lucky to tell it.

On the first day of the trial, Monday, June 7th, 2004, I stopped to get a paper. On the front page of the *Pocono Record* was a story about trial lawyers taking doctors to court in Monroe County without winning a case. The article went on to say that doctors were leaving the state because of these lawsuits. I showed the newspaper to Malcolm and he showed it to the judge. Immediately the judge called the trial lawyers into his chambers. When they emerged, the judge told the jurors to disregard any information in the newspaper.

The jury itself was interesting. Every day for two weeks, they left their families and jobs to sit and listen to this sad story. In Munroe County, there isn't a lot of ethnic difference, not like the bigger cities, and Stroudsburg is a very small city. Still, there were two African American women on the jury and one woman of possibly Indian origin, who wore a sari and a jewel on her forehead. Michael and Malcolm were worried that those three women might not identify with Maureen.

I sat right behind the lawyers during the whole trial with Erik and Ryan beside me. Marcia Kohanski sat beside me too. Lisa followed the trial from home and kept me going emotionally. We watched the lawyers work and the jury's reaction to each piece of evidence and every part of the arguments.

At the outset, Malcolm and Michael showed the jury everything that Maureen went through. They explained the history of the case using Maureen's X-rays, charts and time lines. Marcia organized the medical records so they were in front of the jury day by day. By following the charts, the jury could see the tumors growing through 1994, 1996, and 1997.

Michael and Malcolm then went through the time lines to show every visit to the doctors and the hospitals. The legal staff also created a calendar for the surgeries, chemotherapies, stem cell treatments and radiation. It was all there right up until the day she died, everything Maureen went through: 63 days of chemotherapy, 52 days of stem cell treatment, including 6 days of high-dose chemotherapy, 7 surgeries, and 87 days in the hospital all in one year. The charts were simple, but powerful. The jury took it all in, and they got it.

As the lawyers showed each chart, they asked, "What was the doctor's duty of care? What was the standard of care at this point? Did they do it?" Next to each step on the chart of care procedures was a box to check, *yes* or *no*. After each question the lawyers checked a box. The *no's* added up.

With these exhibits, it was easy for Malcolm and Michael to demonstrate that the three doctors on trial had misdiagnosed Maureen. The same lump in the same spot was finally found to be cancerous. Outside the courtroom, Malcolm kept asking, "Are we missing something?" It all seemed so obvious.

Malcolm explained what happened to Maureen. He told the jury that if she had changed insurance companies earlier, her life might have been saved. With a new insurance company, Maureen changed doctors. This fourth doctor listened to her history, felt the lump, and followed the proper standard of care. Malcolm and Michael showed the jury photographs of Maureen throughout her illness: Maureen in September of 1997, getting ready for stem cell treatment; Maureen in her wig with the boys; Maureen trying to make a 10th birthday for Ryan; Maureen bald and bloated, sleeping on the couch.

Next, Doctor Marie Savard, the prosecution's expert witness, was called to the stand. Dr. Savard is an internist, a women's health expert and a patients' rights champion. Her book, *How to Save Your Own Life: The Savard System for Managing and Controlling Your Healthcare*, tells women to demand their medical records and keep control of them. Before the trial she read Maureen's medical records and they made her angry. Although she doesn't give expert testimony anymore, she did at this trial because the case was so powerful. Dr. Savard's testimony was strong and clear, and Maureen's story is part of her book.

Dr. Savard was convinced that if Maureen had asked for a copy of her mammogram report, Maureen would have asked more questions. Dr. Savard said in her testimony at the trial: "If a patient goes to a doctor and has tests, the patient should not take the doctors word concerning the results. The patient should get a copy of the results and make a binder of the medical records. If Maureen had done so and then gone to another physician, she could have shown the next doctor the other reports. Breast cancer is not treated seriously enough by many doctors in this country. All women are at risk and statistically women of African American descent are at a higher risk. This is very serious."

Doctor Mullen also testified. He told the jury about Maureen's ability to be clear in her medical history, and that she understood the importance of details. She was able to compress the story fast. Dr. Mullen's deposition was essentially a damage deposition, meaning that by the time he started to care for Maureen, all the damage was done. All he could do was help her manage it. Dr. Mullen talked about the failure of her treatment. He said everything they tried didn't work. And it didn't make it any less painful. The stem cell was devastating. He liked Maureen a lot and he is a nice man. All that came through in his testimony.

Malcolm and Michael made sure the jury never forgot Maureen amid all the statistics and technical information. At the end of the day, before the judge let the jury go, they always brought in a witness to talk about Maureen. Their hope was that each juror not just went home thinking about medicine and procedures, but Maureen too. The witnesses at the end of each day were friends and community members who remembered the woman who liked to keep her house clean, take her boys to the mountains, and sit by the pool with her friends. The defense attorneys wouldn't even cross-examine them.

Reverend Steve Sayer was there again for Maureen. Lynn Salerno, Maureen's high school friend from Cranford, New Jersey testified too. She told the jury how she had had a double mastectomy because Maureen had taught her to save her own life.

Helen Sheffo and Laurie Zuchino testified and did a beautiful job. Helen was very upset by the trial; she said it was horrible, reliving Maureen's illness and death. Malcolm wanted her to show the jury the quilts she had made, but the judge wouldn't allow it. Patty Flotz didn't get to testify. She wanted to and she was prepared, but she had to go to Florida for her son's graduation.

And then there was the tape. Right before the trial, Malcolm and Michael asked me if I had more photos, so I brought them everything I could find, including the good-by tape. The first time they heard it they cried: Marcia, Malcolm, Michael, everyone. When they submitted it as evidence, they never expected the judge to allow it. The defense lawyers certainly didn't want the jury to hear it, so they filed all kinds of motions against it.

On the second day of the trial the judge ruled that we could use the tape. When Malcolm played it in the courtroom, everyone froze in place. I couldn't tell if people were breathing. Malcolm talked about the courage it took to sit down and do that. Maureen was so sad and yet she had a complete grasp of what she needed to do. She said, "why me" and she was angry and frustrated, but she regrouped and said, "Erik, be careful don't take such risks, be good to other people. Ryan, I love you." One juror sat with her eyes closed and another juror bent his head, listening to Maureen's words. Many of the jurors watched Erik and Ryan. The boys were hearing their Mom for the first time, speaking to them in front of all these people. The jury understood that Maureen had planned it. Maureen wanted the boys to know nothing could change how much she loved them and now they had witnesses.

The morning before, we were all still at the lawyers' office waiting to hear whether the cassette tape could be used or not. All of a sudden Malcolm started to sing, "Oh what a beautiful morning!" at the top of his lungs. "Oh what a beautiful day!" I thought he'd gone crazy.

"What are you doing?" I asked him.

Michael and Marcia started laughing. "You'd better explain it, Malcolm, or Bill and the boys are going to think we've all lost it."

So Malcolm explained. "Last summer when I went up to Harvard to test this case, it was pretty intense. They video taped the opening and closing arguments and had acting coaches and trial lawyers critiquing and shouting out instructions. 'Back up, look over here, hold your head this way, don't say that.' Lots of other lawyers were using cases they had too. By the second day, we were ragged. We came into this hall, and this great lawyer, Gregory Semano, from Alabama said, 'I think we have some trial lawyers here who are a little beat down. They need some help.' A lawyer from California stood up and started singing, 'Oh what a beautiful morning … there's a bright golden haze on the meadow.' This guy just belted it out, and 72 lawyers sang the refrain, 'Oh what a beautiful morning … everything's going my way.' After that seminar, I went out and bought the soundtrack."

I looked at Malcolm and laughed. "Don't stop singing on account of me." From that time on, when things got tough, we started up that song. I know they sang it together after the boys and I went home. Michael, who should have been an actor, said every night after working sometimes until two in the morning, they'd be going someplace to get something to eat and they'd all be in the car singing that song.

That was the great part, but everyday was still hell, because I was reliving those last months with Maureen fighting for her life. And then there were Maureen's own video taped depositions. The jury watched Maureen answer the lawyers' questions and tell her story. She talked about the stem cell treatments like it was death itself. Even the last tape, when she was only weeks from dying, she remembered dates, medications, treatments and names. At the end of that tape, she removed her wig so everyone could see that she really had lost her hair. She sat with her head up and never took her eyes off the camera. In the span of half a second, she was thirty years older. All the facts and figures became background. Everyone in the courtroom saw Maureen stand up for herself and tell her story.

The last thing she did was smile into the camera for Erik and Ryan even though she had no hair and the circles under her eyes were as dark as charcoal smudges.

Now it was the boys' turn. I didn't really understand until that point how badly they had been hurt. I was too close to it. I couldn't see it. I tried to do everything for them, but watching them on the stand, I realized it hadn't been enough. Erik was 17 now and Ryan was 15. They weren't little kids, they were near men trying to make sense of something they would rather forget. They had lots of questions for the lawyers before trial. Some of their questions I had already answered, but they couldn't understand it then or I was in too much pain to be clear.

Malcolm talked with them to make them understand why we were at trial. They were not happy to be there in the beginning. They didn't get it. Malcolm explained all the things that Maureen had done to keep herself healthy. Then he explained what the doctors had failed to do. He told the boys that their mother didn't deserve what happened to her. When they heard the whole story from Malcolm and when they watched Maureen in the deposition tapes, they understood.

For the first time they had the whole picture. The boys were mesmerized by Maureen in the deposition tapes, and some days they stayed in the office during the trial watching them. There were other reasons for them not to be in the courtroom every day. I didn't want them to go through Maureen's suffering again, and the lawyers said their effect on the jury would be lost if they were there every day. Erik and Ryan also couldn't get enough of the photos. This was them getting to know their mother. We'd go back to the office during a break and Erik would be glued to the T.V. watching the tapes.

Erik was still very guarded and sad. He was the face of anguish and pain. You could see how badly he missed his mother, but he would near say it. Ryan was more open and direct.

Malcolm put Ryan on the stand first.

"Give me a picture of how you imagine or remember your Mom at home," Malcolm asked.

"My favorite things to remember about Mom are how neat everything was and grocery shopping. I used to stand on the rail so she could push her cart. I can still hear her laugh, and I can remember what her voice sounds like. My dad was the tease. He'd tickle me; that was the worst thing. It was fun, but after a while, I'd say, "Mom, make him stop.""

"What else do you remember?"

"I picture her in the house in Bushkill, the only house I ever knew, with her sweatshirt sleeves rolled up, in jeans and in bare feet. I picture her cooking something that smells good. She'd have us climb the apple trees in the yard for apples.

She made pies. She was always involved in school stuff and went on field trips. She'd give the bus drivers cookies. I remember all the camping trips."

"Ryan, do you understand what this trial is about?"

"At first I didn't understand what she was suing about. And the whole trial has been really hard. We had to re-live and hear a lot of stuff. I learned a lot of things. Now I know my Mom should have been treated better."

"What was it like when your mother got sick, Ryan?"

"It sucked." Ryan heard a juror laugh and he said, "Oh, sorry." I don't think the jury minded. He was only telling the truth.

"Do you have any memories of your mother right before she died?"

"In the hospital on Mother's Day, she sang a song by LeAnn Rimes. Something about blue eyes and blue skies. She said, 'I love you Ryan, I'll see you when I get home.' Before she died, I always looked forward to coming home."

"Tell me what you remember about her last day at the house."

"I'll never forget that night. She was screaming, just screaming. I couldn't sleep. I had my pillow over my head. Then my dad came and told us we were going over to the neighbors."

"Tell us what it was like when she died."

"The house got quiet. A lot of it is just a blank part of my life. I don't think you're supposed to remember all that. It was the hardest thing. I remember that. I didn't cry when she died. I was happy she wasn't in pain. She was screaming."

"Who told you that your mother had died, Ryan?"

"I was at the lake when my Dad came and told me. I remember thinking 'what am I going to do now my Mom's gone.' I always thought she was going to come back. I never thought she was going to die. I kept saying I believed she would make it, and I hoped she would. After she died I didn't want to go home. It was quiet, dirty, dark and lonely. Everything stopped, the soccer, the baseball. That was it. It came to an end. I felt lost. I felt like she was the whole world and she was gone."

It was Erik's turn. That morning, as we were driving to the court house, he looked at me and said, "I'm only telling the story once, Dad." He told his story and I learned.

When Malcolm asked him to remember his Mom, Erik answered very clearly. He started talking, looking angry, and Malcolm didn't have to ask him all the questions he had asked Ryan.

"Mom was a shutterbug. Look at all those pictures she took. She was always there. I see her cleaning up or outside if it was nice out. Painting. Always finding something to do and then all of a sudden there was nothing. I was real scared when she got diagnosed with cancer because I had never seen her that way. Dad came to me and said, 'Your mom has cancer and she wants to see you.' My whole world changed that day. Right down to the food in the house. I didn't want to talk about it. I didn't tell my friends. Mainly Ryan and I would go for rides with my Dad and he would explain things. Camping wasn't the same afterwards. It was boring. I don't think we went actually. One year we couldn't go because Dad had to take Mom to the hospital. Me and Ryan went to the community center where everyone was supposed to meet and no one was there. It sucked. They'd already gone.

The first time I thought that she was going to die was when I saw her without her wig at Newton Memorial when she had the stem cell. It really hit me hard.

The last few days before she died were horrible. I couldn't stand the screaming. I wanted to get out of the house and go over to my friend's. I didn't want to go home. I was happier at my friend's house, because it was just too hard. All I could hear was her screaming bloody murder. I was relieved when Mom died. I really missed her, but I didn't want her to be in any more pain. Especially the last few nights, when I realized she wasn't going to make it.

All the trips to the amusement parks, and after a while all the sports, it all stopped. I felt weird, no parents, no rides. Dad was trying to work, and the neighbors didn't want me around. And no more pictures. After she died, the neighbors would send in food. I was embarrassed like we were a charity case.

I felt like the tag-along with the other families, the misfit. Sometimes I would get left at games with no ride home. I didn't want to go over anybody's house anymore because I didn't belong anywhere. It went from coming home and Mom's got cookies and we'd do our homework to coming home to an empty house or Mom's on morphine. Dad tried to save Mom's life. After, there were no more meals around the table. No clean laundry. No one took care of the flowers around the house.

I was in class after Mom died and the teacher actually asked me how she was doing. I said, 'I don't know.' I couldn't even speak. I left class. I just walked out.

I even quit the saxophone after she died even though I had this feeling like I shouldn't. I knew I'd regret it. I was getting in a lot of trouble. I started smoking soon after she got sick. After she died I drank and I got high a lot. It didn't matter. Nothing did."

The courtroom was silent. No one moved when Erik stepped down off the stand. The defense didn't cross-examine either boy.

I was the last witness Malcolm called to testify on behalf of Maureen. Malcolm asked me to talk about Maureen. It was hard to stay focused on Maureen and on my loss and not say anything about the misdiagnosis. I was still so angry, and I wanted Maureen's death to mean something. I wanted to get into the medical information and teach the jury about what women should know so that this would never happen again. I wanted to do the work she would have done if she had survived. But Malcolm told me, "We don't need you to be the doctor. We have an expert. You are the husband and the friend. Tell us about Maureen." I felt like a caged tiger, but Michael and Malcolm knew what they were doing.

Erik and Ryan told the jury what their mom was like, what life was like at our house while she was there. I wanted the jury to know how much I loved Maureen, how she filled my life and how brave she was every minute. I wanted them to know how Maureen faced her death, so I told them about going to see the movie *Titanic*. I saw the jurors cry. I told them how the lights in the theater came up and we were crying and the kids didn't get it and everyone around us was hugging. I told them Maureen knew right then it was over.

Then Malcolm asked me the last question of the prosecution's argument. "Tell us, if you can, what life is like without Maureen?"

I didn't need to think about the answer. "In the six years since Maureen died, I haven't had company. I was with Maureen, sick, for 15 straight months, just care-taking of her. Even then, we enjoyed each other all the time and now I'm alone every day."

On day five of the trial, the defense began their arguments. The defense team was made of at least one lawyer for each of the doctors that was being sued. They were powerful looking as they sat at their table with the doctors sitting behind them. They looked like they owned the courthouse. From the beginning they said it was Maureen's fault that she had cancer. They tried to prove that she missed her mammograms. The defense used Maureen's depositions too. In those tapes they said she was another hysterical woman. They made it look like she worried too much. She was grilled too on why she thought she should get a free mammogram that first time with Dr. Peake. They asked her, "Did you have insurance? Why would you do that? Why did you think you should have a free mammogram?" And there she was on tape in the courtroom, answering every question calmly.

They attacked her character, but gently. Dr. Berger's lawyer was excellent. Dr. Peake's lawyer was a good lawyer too. Dr. Wald's lawyer sometimes blurred the lines of truth. He made subtle attacks. He insinuated that Maureen didn't come back for follow up exams when she was told to, when clearly she had. Or the defense lawyers let the doctors play with the dates; Dr. Berger said, "I expected her to come back in six months and she didn't come back for a year." The truth was the opposite. Maureen had been told to come back in a year and she had gone back in six months. If she came back any earlier, it was because she chose to do it. They were undermining her credibility. The defense lawyers asked the doctors, "Did Mrs. Thiel say in this record that she was doing self-breast examinations?" The question meant, did Maureen report in every office visit that she was doing self-exams at home. If the report didn't make note of it, the defense lawyers tried to establish that she wasn't.

They took advantage of obvious misstatements in the record. They tried to make Maureen look like she wasn't good at remembering dates, or that she wasn't quite truthful. Or maybe the history she gave to Dr. Jackson wasn't quite the same as the one she gave to Dr. Wald. It's pretty difficult for someone to repeat the same history verbatim, over five and a half years. But on the deposition tapes, Maureen did, with only minor variations. She was incredible in every deposition.

At one point, the attorney for Dr. Wald was questioning his client to bring out favorable testimony. He used an example. "Doctor, when you fill out the form, you say Mrs. Whatshername has thus and such, correct?"

I saw Malcolm write something down as soon as he said it. When we got back to the office at lunch break, I asked him what had happened during that testimony.

"We are talking about Maureen, not some theoretical patient. We are all in this courtroom because of Maureen Thiel, not 'Mrs. Whatshername.' It is totally disrespectful!" Malcolm was pacing fast as he talked. "They are going to pay for that mistake."

The primary defense was based on the idea that the doctors could rely on mammograms and ultrasounds to establish a diagnosis. That was the first thing Michael and Malcolm had to overcome, and it was hard. Doctor after doctor they kept hammering away. Michael would ask, "If you have a palpable lump or a cyst beyond thirty days or beyond a cycle, a mammogram or an ultrasound isn't going to tell you anything, is it?" The doctors would have to say, "No." Then they would ask the doctors what the proper standard of care was for a breast lump. Each one of them tried to say they had followed the right standard of care. That was the point Malcolm returned to over and over to beat down the defense. He constantly asked if they relied solely on radiography. They would say, "We relied on the films." And Malcolm would say, "Based on that, you told her everything was O.K?" The answer was always, "Yes."

Dr. Wald's testimony is a good example of how the questioning went, but Dr. Wald had an added twist. Malcolm was ready for him. He walked slowly toward the witness stand, his shoes were polished and his hands clasped loosely in front of his suit coat. Malcolm stopped several feet before the stand and planted his feet firmly at shoulder width.

Dr. Wald did not look at Malcolm at first. He kept his eyes on the back swinging doors of the courtroom. He looked like he was waiting for some minor procedure to end. His suit was gray pin stripe, and he had one leg crossed over the other. Malcolm asked the first question, never taking his eyes off the doctor. "Dr. Wald, you are a successful surgeon, specializing in breast cancer. What tools did you use to establish a diagnosis of Maureen Thiel when she came to you for a surgical consultation?"

At the question, Dr. Wald relaxed slightly, and lifted his chin and as he talked. "I treated her as I treat all my patients. I reviewed her films and took a sonogram of her left breast right there in my office."

Malcolm didn't move. He asked the second question. "So, from looking at her prior mammogram films and taking one sonogram you made a diagnosis. Can you tell us, Doctor, what that diagnosis was and why you were convinced it was correct?"

The smile on Dr. Wald's face grew firmer. He uncrossed his legs and spoke, sometimes pointing directly at Malcolm. "All of the patient's mammograms showed masses and lumps consistent with fibrocystic disease. All of the previous reports indicated that the calcifications were fibrocystic in nature. In the report I sent to Dr. Berger, I did recommend a close watch on some of the architectural abnormalities."

When he stopped, Malcolm leaned his body slightly forward and asked the third question. "Dr. Wald, isn't it true, that there is only one way you could have known whether that was cancer? And that one way is a biopsy, by taking a tiny piece out and putting it on a slide and looking at it? It's the only way. It's been the only way for 200 years and it will be the only way for the next 200 years, until somebody comes up with something different?"

Dr. Wald, tilted his head and pursed his mouth. "Yes, that's true, and I so indicated in my records."

Now Malcolm stepped forward; his hands were loose fists. "Your initial record, Dr. Wald, states nothing of the kind." Malcolm strode back to the prosecution table and retrieved a paper. "Your honor, I would like to introduce into evidence this record from Dr. Wald to Dr. Berger."

"I object!" Dr Wald's lawyer stood and pointed at the paper. "We have already introduced that report into the record."

"Mr. McGregor?" asked the judge.

"Your honor, this record is from Dr. Berger's office. The one the defense has introduced is from Dr. Wald's office. They are not the same record."

"Overruled, and proceed." The judge nodded.

"I would like the court recorder to read back Dr. Wald's testimony of the medical record he kept at his office of Maureen Thiel's visit on May 14th, 1996."

The court recorder read: "Left breast ultrasonography is performed. The left breast is isonated. It is noted that there are multiple areas of architectural distortion in this breast. There are areas of thickened parenchymal tissue as well as cystic appearing areas. These changes appear to be scattered throughout the breast. There is no distinct (i.e. dominant mass) noted. Impression: Multiple architectural distortions, left breast, most likely compatible with fibrocystic disease. Clinical correlation and mammographic correlation are suggested."

"Thank you," said Malcolm. "Now, doctor, would you read to me from this record that we subpoenaed from Dr. Berger's office. Please read the date first."

Dr. Wald went rock still. He took the paper and read. "May 14, 1996. Multiple cysts are noted throughout the left breast. These appear to be simple cysts compatible with fibrocystic disease."

"How is it, Dr. Wald, that there are two different reports? How is that Dr. Berger's report indicates only 'simple cysts' and the report from your office indicates 'thickened parenchymal tissue and architectural distortions'?" How could there be two distinctly different reports for the same visit?"

Dr. Wald's mouth was a very thin line and his eyes went again to the swinging doors at the back of the courtroom. In a tight voice he answered, "I believe it must be a clerical error."

"Or could it be, Doctor, that you altered the records when you heard what had happened to Maureen Thiel?"

"Objection!" yelled his lawyer.

"Sustained," said the judge.

"One more question," said Malcolm quietly. "If, as your report states, you believed Maureen Thiel had abnormalities that you believed required follow up observation, why did she never hear from you again?"

The color came and went from Dr. Wald's face. He opened his mouth to speak, but Malcolm simply stated, "No further questions," and went back to his seat.

Malcolm and Michael could never prove that Dr. Wald had created a "new" original record. Dr. Berger had the original one, but it wasn't the same as Dr. Wald's records. His record had the same date, same patient number, same everything. After he was served with legal papers, he must have looked at the film again and rewritten an interpretation of them. After his testimony, the most powerful attorney from the insurance company, quit the case.

It may sound corny, but it was like Maureen guided us through the trial. Malcolm and Michael both said so. Right from the start, there was a path to take. The records supported her story 100%. Doctor Wald blew her off. He told her she worried too much. He guaranteed her it wasn't cancer, and said, "Don't call us, we'll call you." Malcolm used that line when he cross-examined him. Dr. Wald denied it, and made Maureen out to be a liar, claiming she had never told him about previous visits concerning her breast lump. When Malcolm cross-examined him, it became apparent he remembered things conveniently.

The secondary defense was based on the logic that even if the doctors were wrong for relying on the mammograms and ultrasounds, a biopsy wouldn't have helped, because Maureen had a highly aggressive cancer. By the time the doctors saw her, the cancer was going to kill her anyway. The defense team made a tactical decision to say that the cancer didn't develop until after Maureen had seen Doctors Peake, Berger and Wald.

The defense had an expert witness for malpractice cases. He had a standard testimony: "It was a killer cancer, and would have killed her anyway. It wasn't going to make a difference. Any treatment they had, nothing could handle it." Michael and Malcolm made a list of all the trials where this witness said the same thing. Michael cross-examined him and had the name of each case in which he appeared and the quotation when he testified. Each time it was always almost identical: "It wouldn't have made a difference. The cancer was not related to the condition you treated." Michael went down the list. Finally Michael said, "Well, Doctor Killer Cancer, according to you it would seem that aggressive cancer is entirely out of the realm of diagnosis. None of these doctors were able to identify it in time." The jury loved it. Introducing this logic was an amazingly gutsy, calloused decision on the part of the defense. It defied common sense and totally undermined their credibility.

Michael questioned Dr. Berger. He put his hands in his pockets and rocked back on his heels. "O.K., so what you're saying then is that when Maureen put Dr. Peake's hand on the lump in 1994, it didn't matter, when she went for a mammogram in 1994, it didn't matter, and an ultrasound in 1994, it didn't matter. When she came back in 1995, and you didn't send her for any more tests, it didn't matter. When she came back in 1996 and had mammograms and ultrasounds, it didn't matter. The surgical consultation didn't matter. So everything that she did to try to find her cancer, over two and a half years, didn't matter. This cancer just popped up right before March of 1997 when it was diagnosed. Have I got that right?"

Dr. Berger in her checked, pleated skirt and black wool blazer said, "Yes, that's pretty much what happened. It's just one of those things that can happen sometimes."

Michael stood and looked at the jury to see if they were taking it in. He shrugged his shoulders and said, "No further questions."

I was thrilled to watch Michael and Malcolm beat the snot out of the doctors and lay bare this story. Malcolm told me all along that the goal in the case wasn't just winning. There were smaller goals, such as Maureen being able to give her deposition and tell the truth before she died. Maureen met that goal. File a lawsuit and hold these people accountable, was another goal Maureen met. Making the doctors stand up in court and account for what they did to her was a third goal Maureen met.

Through the entire trial and even before, the defense lawyers never offered a nickel. They defended their case on causation all the way. They defended it saying essentially that the doctors were not negligent, because they have the right to rely on mammograms and ultrasound studies. But even if they were negligent, they didn't cause her cancer; her death was from an aggressive cancer that was going to kill her anyway. They disrespected Maureen, me, Michael and Malcolm. Malcolm kept asking, "Are we missing something?"

At the end Michael's and Malcolm's big concern was the causation issue. They were uncertain if the jury would buy the argument about when the cancer developed and whether Maureen was going to die anyway. Malcolm told me a lot of cases unravel that way. You can get a negligence verdict, but then they say that negligence didn't cause her death.

Michael and Malcolm had asked all the questions and the defense lawyers had had their say. There was nothing left by Thursday afternoon but the closing arguments. The defense lawyers went over the case, saying that Maureen's depositions weren't one hundred percent reliable because she was so sick. They said that the doctors relied on tried and true methods to determine Maureen's condition and that the cancer developed independently of their diagnoses. The defense lawyers repeated that it was an aggressive cancer that would have killed her anyway. Malcolm and Michael were concerned that the jury was going to find the doctors negligent, but not hold them to the cause of Maureen's death.

It was up to Malcolm to explain that Maureen had done everything right. She had led the doctors to her cancer over and over and they neglected to recognize it or to go to the next step and perform the necessary biopsy to determine definitively whether she had cancer or not. She had never been given the proper standard of care and she had been denied not only her first chance but many chances to fight for her life. He told the jury not to listen to the defense arguments. He said. "Look, it is simple what these defense lawyers did here. It's how they defend all these cases and try to deprive the surviving husband and children of their day in court, or give any measure of justice they might have. The lawyers pick up the phone and say, 'We have a case involving Mrs. Whatshername and we need Dr. Killer Cancer.' It's a formula they put together to take to trial. Don't let them do it. The doctors disrespected Maureen Thiel for over two years. Don't let them disrespect Maureen another time."

There was nothing left but for the jury to reach a verdict. At the end of the trial, Malcolm said, "I think we're O.K." But Michael shook his head. "Let's see what happens." In Malcolm's terms, this wasn't a slam dunk case. He told me, "As good as the facts are, as good as it sounds, in Pennsylvania malpractice cases hardly ever win. Physicians are prevailing at a rate of greater than 85%. It's very difficult to win, Bill. Monroe County has not had a malpractice win in over two years, and that settlement was only $40,000. The highest settlement in county history was not over $500,000. Stroudsburg is not a good malpractice town."

Michael and Malcolm both believed the trial had gone as well as they could have hoped.

All the arguments were done on Thursday afternoon. Jury deliberation started right away. We were told to go to Malcolm's office and wait. It didn't seem more than fifteen minutes before we were called back to the courtroom. The jury had a verdict. As soon as he heard it, Malcolm said, "This is not good at all." The jury had decided too fast for Maureen to win. When we sat down in the courtroom, the judge said they couldn't have reached a verdict that quickly, and told them to continue deliberations. We went home.

We all had mixed feelings. On one hand we wanted the trial to be over, on the other hand, we wanted them to decide in Maureen's favor. Michael, Malcolm, Marcia, everyone involved with the case stayed in Stroudsburg over night. During the trial they had moved the whole team to Stroudsburg. They were there for two weeks, away from their families, away from everything. When I asked Malcolm why they did that, why they didn't drive from Scranton every morning, he said, "It gives us a better edge. We get a stronger sense of the trial and of what our clients are going through, the loneliness, the anguish, the pain. You can never reproduce it, but if I went home every night to my kids and my wife, it wouldn't be fair. When you're hearing about someone's loss every day, you're reliving the story, and it gets to you. I don't care who you are, lawyer, judge, you feel it more. I think it makes our work better."

The next morning we reported back to the courthouse and checked in with the judge and then went to the office in Stroudsburg. We were all tense, even the boys, when Malcolm started the song. Michael and Marcia joined in, and they made the boys and me sing too. Michael got up on the table and acted out the horse and buggy. We were all belting out, "Oh what a beautiful morning" at the top of our lungs. The window was open and people stopped on the street.

From there Michael and Malcolm started telling funny trial stories. They were playing around, trying to keep everybody hopeful. Erik and Ryan asked how the verdict worked, because they wanted the doctors' licenses taken away and the doctors to go to jail. They were angry. Malcolm said it was possible the doctors could lose their licenses, but they wouldn't go to jail.

We were in the conference room talking, and I looked around at everyone. I got tears in my eyes thinking about how much this legal team had given me and Maureen. "I love you guys," I said. Michael and Malcolm stopped clowning and looked at me. I didn't realize until that moment what was involved in making a case go. When it all came together, I was amazed. I felt so close to those guys at that moment and I knew Maureen was right there with us.

We all jumped when the phone rang. It was the courthouse telling us the jury was finished. It had only been another hour and a half of deliberations. Michael's face was serious when he put down the phone. Malcolm took me aside and said, "Bill, I don't think this is good news. Even though the case went well, when there's a quick verdict, it means they haven't assessed the damages and they find in favor of the doctors. You've been classy throughout this whole trial and I don't want you to show any emotion now."

I understood. "It's not going to change me and I'm so grateful for all you've done. I'm sorry that if it isn't successful for all your hard work.

"We'll see," was all he answered.

As we walked over, Malcolm and Michael kept asking, "What else could we have done? Where did we miss something?" Michael said again, "It's never good news when a jury comes back this quickly." We sat in the courtroom and waited. All the defense lawyers were there. They came over and commended us on a job well done. Doctors Peake and Wald were there, but Doctor Berger wasn't. Malcolm thought it was the final act of disrespect for Maureen.

Malcolm and Michael were convinced it was a defense verdict right up until the jury walked in. They told me later they read the body language and it looked good; almost all the jurors looked at us except for two.

I looked at the jury and thought about how Maureen wanted them to know what had happened. She had done her job. She had been in that room talking to all of us. No matter what happened, she had made it this far. I remembered the scream and I remembered making the promises. And then I remembered her dark, curly hair on Sand Key Beach as she stood in front of the waves and the late afternoon sun. I remembered her eyes so full of fun. I didn't need the jury to tell me anything.

The judge, very solemn, said, "Do you have a verdict?" The foreman stood up. He handed the verdict to the judge. In a malpractice suit in Pennsylvania the case is stated in a two-part question. For the defendants to be found guilty, the answers have to be *yes* and *yes*. The judge asked the first question, "Do you find that the defendant, Dr. Peake was negligent in the standard of care for breast cancer?" If the jury didn't answer that question with *yes*, we were done. We held our breath. The foreman said, loud enough so there was no mistake, *No.* The judge asked the same question for Doctor Berger. The answer came back *Yes* and *Yes* again for Doctor Wald.

I said, "Oh, my God!" out loud.

"What, Dad, what?" Erik was pulling on my arm. I put my hand up to tell him to wait.

The next question was about causation. That was the basis of their defense. If the jury agreed that the cancer was aggressive anyway, then they would decide that the doctors had not increased Maureen's risk of harm. The judge asked the final question: "Did the actions of the defendant, the negligent defendants

Doctor Berger and Doctor Wald, increase the risk of harm so that Maureen Thiel would die and thus caused her death?" Not only did our breath stop, but there was no blood moving in our veins. Everyone was like stone. *Yes,* came the answer from the foreman.

I saw Michael and Malcolm flinch. We were all staring at the jury, waiting to hear the damages they believed we should receive. "We find in favor of the plaintiff in the amount of $5.4 million dollars."

Malcolm actually shuddered. Michael bowed his head. Marcia started crying. We all started crying. And hugging. Everybody. At that instant, it all came together. These lawyers knew the importance of this story, and it touched them like no other case in the history of their firm had ever touched them.

Maureen was vindicated. She was respected. These people understood what she went through and everything she had done. She had guided us. Those two lawyers held each other and cried because the jury believed Maureen. I was just numb.

"What happened, Dad? What happened?" Erik and Ryan said together.

I started crying at the sound of their voices. "Mom won. Your Mom won." I grabbed them in my arms and hugged them the way Maureen would have.

Everyone was leaving the courtroom, Erik and Ryan walked out with Marcia, but I sat back down. I sat with my head in my hands trying to take it in.

"Bill, they're waiting for you." It was Michael, calling me into the hall.

"What?"

"The jury is outside waiting for you."

"Why?"

"They want to talk to you."

The jury wanted to give Erik, Ryan and me their condolences, because they were so appalled by Maureen's story. Ten jurors were waiting in the hall. Michael said he had never seen that happen before. One or two jurors, maybe, but not ten.

They hugged me and said what a strong woman Maureen was, and they were so sorry. I saw the compassion in their eyes. During my drives to the courthouse, I thought about what the jurors were going through. I thanked them for listening to this hard story.

It was the women who asked to speak to me, especially the African American women, a Caucasian woman and the Indian woman. A Muslim woman, who wore a head scarf through the whole trial, was like a heat seeking missile. She zeroed in on Erik. Through the trial this woman had watched Erik and Ryan. She could see the sadness and anger in Erik. Ryan was hurting too, but Erik was contorted inside. This woman pulled Erik aside and said, "We have given you your mother's revenge. Now you must go on with your life." She looked him dead in the eye and told him that. She knew he needed to hear that it was time for him to let go. It's no accident that he became sober and closer to Ryan and me after that.

I thanked them all. Michael and Malcolm stood back and watched. Those jurors told us, "We can't take away what happened to you, but we can let you know we agree it was wrong. Maureen was right."

Then the jurors told me that they had wanted to award the estate $20 million dollars, but they were worried it would be appealed and the boys would have to wait. Then they thought maybe $10 million, but again that was a pretty big number. There might be appeals and the insurance companies might not pay it, but they thought $5.4 million might work. But it didn't matter, because the amount of the settlement had been agreed upon before the verdict was read. As is the case in most medical malpractice cases, Maureen got far less in her estate than the jury wanted her to have. And that didn't matter either. This case was never about the money. It was always about getting at the truth.

Maureen's estate got enough to pay the attorney's fees and expenses. The state statute sets a portion aside for the children and the remainder I have used to fund this book, the website and all fund raising activities to get this story told. I was not in control of who got what.

Michael and Malcolm got calls from lawyers all over the state because the verdict award was of such magnitude. Across the United States the percentage of 5 million dollar verdicts is miniscule. In Pennsylvania the percentage is even smaller. In Monroe County it's not even on the radar. That's the power of this story.

The jury even told us that when they deliberated on Thursday they very quickly came to a plaintiff's consensus. But two women were opposed. One woman came the next day with breast cancer data to try and sway the rest of the jurors. Bringing data outside of the evidence is illegal, so the other jurors threatened to get sheriff. Those two women wouldn't give up their vote, so it was ten to two.

Doctor Wald was in the hall too. He asked Malcolm if he could apologize not for anything he did, but for how sorry he was for our loss.

I told Malcolm I didn't know if I was ready for that. Malcolm didn't blame me and told Dr. Wald that now was not the time. When Dr. Wald walked by, he caught my arm as I was turning away from the jury. He reached out and said, "I'm really sorry for the loss of your wife."

My "Thank you," came out automatically, like when someone says "God bless you when you sneeze.

I stood there, not believing it was over. We walked back to the law office, and then I said to Erik and Ryan, "C'mon, let's go see your Mom." Everyone else came too. We all drove to Maureen's grave, because that's were we belonged. We went there to be with Maureen.

Malcolm heard *Stairway to Heaven* on the radio on the way there. When I thanked them for coming, Marcia said, "This was Maureen's battle, it wasn't ours. We were just carrying out her wishes. We needed to come here and tell her."

But the truth was, when we got there, we all knew the same thing: Maureen already knew. She was there. We all felt her presence. And it wasn't just that the dogwood tree next to her grave had finally flowered for the first time, six years after she died.

Chapter Seven

Maureen's Mission

The trial and the verdict were an ordeal and a triumph. It was everything Maureen had wanted it to be. Erik and Ryan would be taken care of and the doctors had been publicly held accountable. The state investigated the doctors after the trial was over. That's never happened after a case the Foley law firm tried. After the boys were awarded their share in the trust, I used the money I received to do what Maureen wanted. Now I didn't have to worry how I was going to feed the kids every month. From that money, I gave 10% to church, and it helped the community build a new church. That was always part of Maureen's wish. She was real firm that that was going to happen. Maureen was always clear that she was going to make a significant gift, and that says something about her faith, about her commitment, about what she thought was important. A lot of people sue each other just to make a buck.

But all of that was between Maureen and me. I guess once Maureen was gone I could have put the money in my pocket. We didn't have anything in writing, just what we decided together. I have honored her every step of the way.

The trial had benefits that went beyond money. Erik and Ryan understood better what they had suffered and why they had suffered it. They had a lot of guilt and blamed themselves, like most kids do. It's part of grief. They also realized that someone else killed her. It lifted a weight off them. Malcolm and Michael talked very honestly to them. The boys were smoking pot, drinking, even doing stronger drugs. The lawyers didn't try to lecture, but reminded them of what Maureen had said on the tape. Marcia made them each a copy, and Malcolm told them, "I would treasure that. That's your mother captured in time for the rest of your life, wishing you life's blessings and good will, and trying to protect you from the grave. You have to think before you make choices about how you betray those words." It made an impression on Erik and Ryan.

They're good kids, but they were lost and sad. Ryan started drawing after she died, and that helped him through a lot. After the trial, he became even more serious about his art. Several months after the trial, I brought Erik to the Clear Brook Detoxification Center. He's been sober ever since, and he started college several months after that. Malcolm and I still have a nice relationship. He does with the boys too. Erik's off to college, because Malcolm and Michael helped find the right school for him to attend. The boys also have copies of all the deposition tapes. They want to put them together and make a video of the parts where Maureen isn't talking about cancer, the nicer parts. That's all they have of that year.

Maureen and I were definitely two peas in a pod. We were soul mates, if there is such a thing. But I had to get on with my life. Now I have Lisa, and she's amazing. I don't compare Lisa to Maureen. Lisa sat through the whole trial and knows that Maureen is a part of me. Not every woman could do that. The boys are fairly well adjusted now, because they've learned to live their lives without their mother. I'm there for them now, and I love them the way Maureen asked me to.

At some point in all this I realized that I had been feeling too sorry for myself. That was the day I became human again. Some people stay in that role and never come back out. Maureen was definitely the instigator, the planner in our marriage. I was so in love with her, I did whatever she needed me to do. Now I had to plan for myself.

Only a few hours after Maureen's trial the *Pocono Record* wanted to interview me. The reporter started with, "Let me first ask, how does it feel to be a millionaire, are you going to retire?" I had no words for this question. I had just been through a trial that crushed me. I managed something rude and hung up the phone. I called Malcolm and Malcolm called the paper. A few hours later I received an apology and we went on to do the interview. The next morning I got the paper only to read, *$5.4 Million Verdict*, as the headline. (*Pocono Record*, June, 2004) The story was all about the verdict, and very little about what I had told them, very little about what I promised Maureen. In the article it said that Maureen's breast cancer was misdiagnosed by her doctors due to a delayed biopsy. Everyone read the verdict, but no one cared about the misdiagnosis.

It has been over two years since the trial, and not one person from the media has called me to ask, "Bill, could anything have been done to prevent the misdiagnosis? Is there any way to prevent it from happening again?" Over the next few weeks I began the second part of my promise. I new what my commitment would be for the rest of my life.

Gill Garrett from *Health Watch 16 News* gave me the first opportunity. She took me seriously, and she didn't care about the verdict. She cared about the story and how important it was to get the message across. In September 2004, WNEP-TV Channel 16's *Health Watch* out of Scranton, Pennsylvania did a story. They have about 104,000 viewers. A month later, they did a follow up on their main news report. That was it. All the reporting was done as far as the media was concerned.

All this time, during the six years leading up to the trial, I was still contacting people at the *American Cancer Society* and the *National Breast Cancer Foundation* to ask them why our doctors didn't follow the *American Medical Association* Standard of Care. I talked with people at the *Susan G. Koman Breast Cancer Foundation*. No one could give me answers. I asked for answers and the more questions I asked the more I understood what the real questions should be. I made phone calls every day. I emailed people every day. I did that because every time I told Maureen's story, someone said, "Oh, I had a lump too and they told me not to worry." Or, "I had a friend who had a lump and it wasn't until she insisted on a biopsy that they found out it was cancer." I kept asking because I didn't ever want to hear another story like Maureen's.

While the trial was going on, everyone was under a gag order; I couldn't talk to anybody about the case or tell the story. Once the verdict came in, I was free. I talked to everybody I met about Maureen's story. But what more could I do? It was over. Why couldn't that just be good enough? Why couldn't I stop right there? But it wasn't over. I couldn't stop, because of the promises I made to Maureen. The first and most important thing to Maureen was to finish this lawsuit. Second, it was important to get her story out. Maureen wanted to save women's lives. If she could have gotten on the Oprah Show, she would have felt like a success.

The promise I made to Maureen was bigger than any trial settlement. At the trial, when they played Maureen's first deposition before she had the stem cell treatment, I heard her saying how she was going to talk to other women about what she had been through. "I'm going to be an advocate, if I make it," she said. Those words came back to me, over and over.

The first time I watched it I didn't cry. I was stunned and paid attention. At the end of the video, Maureen voiced her concern about women she was never going to meet. She wanted to warn women. The more I watched that tape, the madder I got until I was as mad as Maureen the day of the scream, the scream that kills me when I close my eyes and hear it. That scream has never gotten any softer. I guess Maureen meant it to be that way, because it keeps me focused.

I knew I had to tell her story every day. While I was on my Fed Ex route, I told her story. When I met someone at the store, I told her story. When I went to the dentist, I told her story. Every time, someone would say, "You should write a book."

Why would I want to write a book about what we went through? Why would I relive all that horror and pain? Would it heal me? Am I ever going to heal? Probably not. But I had to move on and this was the only way I could move forward. I contacted authors on the Internet. I spoke with a few and even had one or two start writing, but nothing felt right. Then I contacted a writer named Pat Schneider, in Amherst, Massachusetts. She writes poetry, novels, plays, and lyrics. She also leads writing workshops. She gave me the names of three writers that she thought might work out for me. I'm sure I spoke with all of them, but it was when I talked to Maureen Buchanan Jones, that I knew we were a match. We talked on the phone two or three times and I drove to her house. I brought Maureen's and my photo albums, newspaper clippings, Maureen's medical records, and five cassette tapes I had made telling the story. This book began with me talking into a tape recorder and Maureen Buchanan Jones listening very hard.

I knew that wasn't going to be enough. The more I thought about it, the bigger the promise I made to Maureen became. Maureen wouldn't have been satisfied either. She would have kept going, so I kept going. I wish Maureen could tell this story in her own way, but she is my angel guiding me in the right direction. She was still trying to leave her mark on people's hearts (*Pocono Record* May 17, 2005).

The promise she asked me to keep was one of the hardest things I've ever done in my life, but it is worth all the pain of not letting her go. Maureen knew I would be proud to tell her story and each time the pain would be replaced with gratitude, love and honor to fulfill her promise. I am more proud of Maureen than ever before. She is a survivor; maybe not in her own body, but in the way she wanted to survive, by letting everyone know what happened to her. If one woman listens to Maureen's story and gets a correct, early diagnosis, then Maureen has won with them.

Now I've taken on the mission to help end misdiagnosis in this country. I created *Maureen's Mission*, a non-profit organization to educate women on the standards of care in diagnosing and treating a breast lump. (*Citizens Voice* news article, May 17, 2005) I founded *Maureen's Mission* with the help of Malcolm MacGregor and Michael McDonald, the lawyers who tried Maureen's lawsuit and with the help of Paul Lyon, the Executive Director of the *Committee for Justice for All*. I established a website at www.maureensmission.org. To kick off *Maureen's Mission* I held a press conference at the Victoria Inn and Conference Center in Pittston, Pennsylvania where I announced not only the launch of the *Mission*, but a fund-raising event. I organized a golf tournament at the Four Seasons Golf Club in Exeter, Pennsylvania for May 28th of 2005. I invited the media, and the following stations and newspapers covered the story: WNEP TV; WBRE TV; the *Citizens Voice, Times Leader, Sunday Dispatch, Times Tribune* and the *Morning Call* newspapers. Their viewers and readers number about 350,000.

On the day of the tournament more press came. WNEP TV and WBRE TV both covered my "Swing for Life" Golf Outing Fundraiser with estimated viewers at 154,000. Not long after, Lyndell Stout, Co-anchor of WBRE-TV's Channel 28 Main News Program, interviewed me on *The Buddy Check-Up*. The estimated viewing audience was 40,000 in Wilkes Barre, Pennsylvania.

In the months that followed, I called, emailed and knocked on doors. I did television and radio interviews. I wrote pieces for web sites that covered breast cancer news, and newspapers followed developments in the story. In November of 2004, I appeared on *Defining Women* a radio talk show on WMRD 1420-AM, out of Middletown, Connecticut. Estimated listeners 117,000. In April of 2005, I was the guest speaker at the Horizon of Hope Fundraiser, in Dallas, Pennsylvania, at the Irem Temple Golf and Country Club. One hundred people attended. *Women's Forum*, a web magazine covered Maureen's story with over 8 million readers daily. The *Young Women's Survival Coalition*, another web magazine published a piece on Maureen; their readership is about 2.5 million daily. The *Y-Me Organization*, out of Chicago, Illinois, also ran an article that I wrote. Two million people visit their website daily. In September 2005, I appeared on WVIA TV, a local affiliate of PBS, on a talk show, *State of Pennsylvania*, produced by Susan Kelly. It's a one-hour show out of Pittston, Pennsylvania with estimated viewers at 256,000.

By October of 2005, I was busy. WILK Radio, also in Pittston, Pennsylvania, invited me for their one-hour talk show with estimated listeners at 220,000. I was the guest speaker before 100 people at the Women's Health Insurance Commission of Susquehanna Valley, Bloomsburg, Pennsylvania. A Channel 61 talk show included me in their production, as well as the talk show, *Corner4Success*, out of Las Vegas, Nevada, with 400,000 estimated listeners.

But I wasn't satisfied with just the press getting the word out. I knew there was something fundamentally missing from the story. I kept going back to Maureen's scream and knew that I never would have heard it if someone had educated us about the proper steps to follow once Maureen found the breast lump. Based on a lot of research, I wrote an educational pamphlet called *If You Find a Lump: What Every Woman Should Know*. I created this pamphlet from direct quotes and guidelines from many organizations. One of the best resources for this pamphlet was Doctor Lillie Shockney, RN, BS, MAS, Administrative Director of the *Johns Hopkins Avon Foundation Breast Center* in Baltimore, Maryland. I visited Johns Hopkins and spoke with her for several hours, and she gave me vital information.

I drafted this pamphlet as a way to convey the necessary information to any woman who has just found a breast lump. If Maureen and I had been handed information like this, we never would have listened to the doctors, and we would have followed the correct guidelines to ensure an early, correct diagnosis. A pamphlet like this still doesn't exist today. This pamphlet is being circulated to some of the best breast care organizations in the country for their opinion and advice. Many breast cancer coalitions in other states have agreed to give their input. Once this pamphlet is perfected, I will seek to have it endorsed by as many credible people in the field of breast care as I can. My prayer is that one day it will be mandated that every woman with a breast lump will be handed this pamphlet. It will be every woman's right to be educated in her diagnosis, treatment and follow-up of her breast concern. Every woman will know the guidelines.

I brought a draft of this pamphlet to Pennsylvania Representative, Phyllis Mundy and Calvin Johnson, the Pennsylvania Secretary of Health (*Times Leader*, "Man Takes Mission to Harrisburg"). Secretary Johnson agreed that women need more education. Both he and Representative Mundy have advised me on the pamphlet. After months of research, using thousands of documents, I have condensed the necessary information for the contents of the pamphlet. The Secretary of Health stated that if the pamphlet is based on credible resources and is endorsed by reputable medical sources, he will review it and propose a mandate that all women in the state of Pennsylvania receive this pamphlet when a breast lump is found.

On the following page is the pamphlet that I have drafted. It is to be used as an aid in guiding diagnosis and treatment.

What Every Woman Should Know.

Breast lumps

- Breast lumps, cysts or other breast abnormalities are common in all women.
- Approximately 85 % of all breast lumps are benign (non-cancerous).
- Breast disease is not a death sentence, but a misdiagnosis can be life threatening.
- All lumps/masses/cysts should be treated as cancerous until proven benign for your safety.
- If you are pre-menopausal, breast lumps are usually caused by hormonal changes.
- If you find a lump, or your doctor finds one during a clinical evaluation or any diagnostic testing, speak with your doctor about it.

Specialization

- Breast care requires specialized attention, just as the heart or lungs do.
- Make sure that your health care provider is specialized in breast care.
- If your health care provider is not specialized in breast care, you have the right to be referred to a breast care center that specializes in breast care.
- If, because of where you live, you cannot receive treatment at a breast care center, ask to have the results of all imaging studies sent to a breast care center and reviewed before a diagnosis is made.
- Do not depend on a health care provider who is not specialized in breast care.
- Ask your radiologist if he or she is specialized; most radiologists prefer a second opinion if they are not specialized.

Team Work

- Your doctor and radiologist will answer all your questions and include you in decisions based on the results of your imaging studies.
- Therefore you, your personal doctor, your radiologist and surgeon, all specialized in breast care, will work as a team for your safety and to ensure a correct diagnosis.

Education

- Educate yourself for your safety. Ask to view your films with your doctor; it is your responsibility to understand what is in your breast.
- Get a copy of the patient guidelines for breast care from the ACS, the NCI, or the NCCN. Read them, follow them, know them and understand them.
- If your health care providers can't answer your questions, find ones who can.
- Keep all medical records; ask any questions you think are necessary. Take someone with you to medical appointments to help remember questions, listen to answers and take notes. You may also bring a tape recorder.

Guidelines

- Guidelines to diagnosing breast disease and breast abnormalities are available from your health care provider, from the NCCN, NCI, the ACS, or www.guidelines.gov.
- Follow these guidelines to ensure the highest quality care for your breast abnormality. With these guidelines you will know what symptoms and conditions cause concern and are agreed upon by doctors and radiologists in diagnosing and treating your breast abnormality.

Early Diagnosis

- A diagnosis should be made within 4-6 weeks of the initial discovery of the lump.
- Women correctly diagnosed with breast cancer in its early stages have a higher cure rate and a higher survival rate.

Exams/Biopsies

- Call your doctor if you find any abnormality. A breast self exam(BSE), clinical breast exam (CBE), mammograms and ultrasounds can detect abnormalities, but a biopsy is the only procedure that shows whether a mass is cancerous or not.
- Your physician will evaluate your breast changes using a combination of a physical breast examination, mammography, and an ultrasound and/or biopsy.
- Although none of these are 100% accurate, when combined, they are usually successful at diagnosing your condition correctly.
- Once a breast abnormality has been found, you should expect the following steps in diagnosing the abnormality:
  1. Clinical exam,
  2. Mammogram, Ultrasound or both, depending on your age. An ultrasound can be the first and only test required, if your specialist recommends it and you are under 30 years of age.
  3. Biopsy, if recommended by radiologist.

Biopsy

- Not all breast lumps need a biopsy.
- It is important to remember that all breast abnormalities do not require a biopsy, but all abnormalities should be treated seriously until a definite diagnosis is made.
- There are many types of biopsies. Your doctor and radiologist will explain them to you. It is up to you to understand and be part of the decision as to what type of biopsy is best for you.
- An ultrasound-guided or stereotactic, x-ray needle biopsy, performed by a radiologist specialized in this procedure is one type of biopsy that may be recommended.
- Or your doctor may recommend a surgical biopsy, performed by a surgeon specialized in breast care.
- If you are anxious and want to know without a doubt if you have breast cancer, it is your right to demand a biopsy.
- A biopsy is the only tool that can tell you if a lump/mass/cyst is cancerous or not.

Diagnosis

- A correct diagnosis is imperative.
- The following steps are necessary to complete the diagnostic process:
  1. A biopsy/aspiration has established the diagnosis of benign breast conditions.
  2. A biopsy/aspiration has established the presence of malignancy.
  3. Both patient and doctor agree the lump has completely disappeared.
- If you are a woman with a history of common cysts, your doctor may recommend that you wait until after your menstrual cycle to see if your lump will dissipate. If, after your menstrual cycle, the lump persists, go back to your doctor.
- If you are menopausal, don't wait; get every lump checked by your doctor.
- If your team of breast care providers believes that your lump is a common cyst or other common abnormality, a biopsy may not be recommended.
- If your lump has dissipated or shrunken you will be told to schedule your follow-up appointments according to the guidelines set forth by the American Cancer Society.
- It is your responsibility to return for a follow-up after one menstrual cycle if recommended. Returning for your follow-up will ensure you of an early diagnosis.
- The preferred option for evaluating a dominant mass is to proceed directly to an ultrasound, Which is performed by a radiologist specialized in breast imaging.
- If the ultrasound evaluation reveals that the mass is consistent with an asymptomatic simple cyst, the abnormality may be observed without an aspiration or biopsy.
- If your lump persists for more than one menstrual cycle, an aspiration or biopsy should be performed. A radiologist, based on the results of mammograms and ultrasounds, may recommend a biopsy as the next step.
- Other symptoms or your level of anxiety may also be good reasons to recommend a biopsy.
- The American Cancer Society recommends that all suspicious lesions undergo aspiration/biopsy to rule out neoplasm and to obtain a definite diagnosis.
- The American Society in the *Patient Guidelines Version VI/September 2004 Breast Biopsy*, states: "If a woman or her doctor finds a suspicious

breast lump, dominant mass, lesions or if imaging studies show a worrisome area, the women must have a biopsy."

- Your team of doctors can make and confirm a final diagnosis when the clinical evaluation, mammographic studies and/or ultrasounds and pathological studies from the biopsy all agree. From the diagnosis, treatment options will be discussed and recommended.
- It is important that you are comfortable with the diagnosis and that all abnormalities have been proven benign (non-cancerous).

More women are diagnosed with breast cancer today than ever before. But mortality rates have declined, thanks to the efforts of many organizations. While these organizations seek to eradicate breast cancer, breast cancer is still claiming lives.

The information in this pamphlet is not recognized as an official, medical standard of care, but it is based on credible sources. Your health care provider, specialized in breast care, is your best source of knowledge for your diagnosis.

The following questions are typical when a woman has found a lump in her breast:

Question: I found a lump or have a change in my breast, what do I do?
Answer: Call your doctor for an appointment to get a clinical exam.

Question: I was told after mammograms and an ultrasound that I have simple cysts, not to worry about them, and to come back in 6 months or a year for a follow-up. Should I be satisfied with that information?
Answer: No. The guidelines set forth by many organizations require you, the patient, to return after one menstrual cycle, or within 30 days to have a lump re-evaluated. If it is a simple cyst, it can dissipate on its own. If the lump persists, further evaluation must be done to ensure correct diagnosis. An aspiration or a biopsy is the only way to be sure a persistent lump is not cancerous.

Question: I've asked my doctor if she specializes in breast care and she told me she does not. What should I do?
Answer: Ask for a referral to a breast care center immediately. If you are unable to go to a breast care center, have your file sent to a center for diagnosis.

Question: Where do I get the guidelines for breast cancer and breast disease?
Answer: You can get them online from the websites for the NCCN, the NCI, the AMS, or at www.guidelines.gov.

Question: When do I know I have the correct diagnosis?
Answer: When you have ruled out cancer 100%, or you have been told after a biopsy that you have a malignancy.

Question: Where else can I get credible information immediately?
Answer: You can get many questions answered online or at *Ask an Expert* at the Johns Hopkins Avon Breast Care Center: www.hopkinsbreastcenter.org/servcies/ask_expert. This site is highly recommended and is one of the leaders in the field of breast care. Also the NCI, the NCCN, the NCI, the AMS, the Y-ME Organization, the Susan G. Komen Organization., and the Young Survival Coalition all have links to helpful resources.

Question: I have no access to a computer, where can I go for all this information?
Answer: Your health care provider has access to all this information. Ask him or her for the guidelines. He or she should be glad to help. Remember, you are part of a team; everyone is working together to help you with a correct diagnosis.

Question: My doctor makes me feel like I am not allowed to be part of the team, and hesitates to give me information. What should I do?
Answer: Go to another health care provider and tell them of your circumstances. Breast disease and breast abnormalities have become a specialized field. When abnormalities occur, the process of making a diagnosis must incorporate everyone as a team especially you, the patient.

Question: How do I find a breast specialist?
Answer: Your own doctor may be specialized in breast care. It is important to ask him/her. They should refer you to a breast specialist if they are not. If you need a referral, there are resources to help you. Local hospitals and medical schools have lists of breast specialists. State, county and city medical societies know who among them are specialized in breast care. Local divisions of the American Cancer Society (ACS) are a source. The National Cancer Institute, (NCI); the Y-ME, a leader among Breast Cancer Support Organizations; and Johns Hopkins Avon Breast Care Center are among the

best resources for information. There are many other great resources for information on finding a breast specialist. Treatment from a breast specialist can mean an early, correct diagnosis rather than a delayed, life-threatening misdiagnosis. Give yourself the best chance and the best knowledge. You deserve it.

This educational pamphlet, created by *Maureen's Mission,* is the result of a promise made to Maureen Thiel to help save women's lives. If Maureen Thiel had read this pamphlet when she first found a lump, she might be alive today. The information in this pamphlet is borrowed by permission from The National Comprehensive Cancer Network (NCCN), The National Cancer Institute (NCI), the American Cancer Society (ACS), Intracorp, Philadelphia, PA., and The Frontier Health Care.

Further resource material:
> *Breast Cancer Screening and Diagnosis Guidelines* (NCCN)
> *Breast Cancer, Treatment Guidelines for Patients* (NCCN, ACS)
> *Breast Masses* (Intracorp, 2005 Philadelphia, PA.)
> *Breast Cancer* (ACS)
> *Early Diagnosis of Breast Abnormalities* (Frontier Healthcare)

Through *Maureen's Mission* I am also working to get legislation that would create standards in diagnosing, treating and following up a breast lump. Currently there are none. I was told by doctors that the standard of care in a diagnosis can vary from one side of the street to the other. I was also told that we are years away from such a standard being universally recognized. Millions of dollars are spent writing guidelines and doing research in breast care, but no doctor is mandated to follow them.

I can accept that my wife died of breast cancer, but I will never accept that she was misdiagnosed. No woman in this country should ever be misdiagnosed. I'm working hard to end it and so is Senator Jane C. Orie. On Thursday, July 21, 2005, I brought to Senator Orie a legislative bill that could change the way women receive care for breast concerns. Senator Orie supports this bill and is helping to put it before the Pennsylvania legislature. This bill will create a clearer path for early, correct diagnoses. All women in this country deserve *The Breast Care Center Treatment Act*. This bill would ensure that all women have access to a specialized health care provider in breast care. If a woman, because of geographic location, cannot get treatment from a health care provider specialized in breast care, then her health care provider must forward her file to a specialized health care provider before a diagnosis can be made. Before the bill can pass, a resolution has been put before the legislature. This resolution was drafted by Senator Orie and me and was introduced to the Pennsylvania State Legislature in July 2006, just before this book was published. It reads as follows:

A Resolution Directing the Joint State Government Commission to Create a Pink Ribbon Advisory Committee to Study the Timely Detection of Breast Cancer

WHEREAS, many women in Pennsylvania are continuing to live a normal life because of early detection of breast cancer; and

WHEREAS, many women have been afforded the opportunity to undergo screening for breast cancer; and

WHEREAS, the combination of detection through screening and treatment with more effective therapies has prolonged the lives of women diagnosed with breast cancer through screening; and

WHEREAS, there are women who, despite screening, have succumbed to cancers that were not detected in their early stages; and

WHEREAS, Pennsylvania is desirous of increasing the incidence of early detection of breast cancer so that more of the Commonwealth's women may live out their normal life spans; and

WHEREAS, Pennsylvania, with its many medical schools, teaching hospitals, and world renowned cancer specialists and breast surgeons and cancer and breast centers, is fortunate to have the expertise available to recommend what may be done to increase the incidence of early detection of breast cancer; therefore be it

RESOLVED, that the Senate direct the Joint State Government Commission to conduct a study on the timely detection of breast cancer; and be it further

RESOLVED that, at a minimum, the Joint State Government Commission study (1) the state of breast cancer screening technology; (2) the cost of that technology; (3) the education and training of those who perform the screening and interpret the results; (4) the numbers of qualified breast imaging or mammography radiologists; (5) the numbers of screening and treating professionals and paraprofessionals in relation to the numbers of women in the Commonwealth; (6) the accessibility of women in rural areas to the professionals and paraprofessionals; (6) the existence of guidelines for breast imaging or mammography; (7) the incidence of adherence to the guidelines; (8) the existence of and adherence to guidelines for follow-up with women found to have abnormal symptoms; (9) the need to create a Pennsylvania guideline or standard of care for detection and fol-low-up; (10) the adequacy of provider reimbursement by both the public and pri-vate sector; (11) the availability of insurance for first and second opinions; and (12) the information made available to women who have been found to have abnormal symptoms; and be it further

RESOLVED, that the Joint State Government Commission create a Pink Ribbon Advisory Committee composed of individuals from Breast Centers, from Cancer Centers; rural breast and cancer centers; from breast imaging radiologists, breast surgeons, primary care providers, including family practitioners and obstetrical-gynecologists; mammography/breast imaging technologists; the administration of facilities which perform mammography and imaging technol-ogy; and the insurance industry ; and representatives of advocacy groups such as the Pennsylvania Breast Cancer Coalition, and the Susan B Komen Foundation; and from representatives of any other interested parties the Commission shall choose to assist it in its deliberations; and be it further

RESOLVED, that the Commission provide the Senate with its findings and rec-ommendations on how Pennsylvania can increase the incidence of detecting breast cancer; and be it further

RESOLVED, that the Commission report its findings and recommendations to the Senate no later than one year from date of enactment.

My hope is that once the study is complete, the Bill printed below will pass the Pennsylvania Legislature to enforce the proper standard of care for all women in this state.

THE GENERAL ASSEMBLY OF PENNSLVANIA

HOUSE BILL

No. 2355 Session of 2005

Introduced by: William C. Thiel

THE BREAST CARE CENTER TREATMENT ACT

To ensure all women have the right to be treated at a breast care center for the diagnosis, treatment, and follow-up of a breast abnormality, or have their records sent to a breast care center for diagnosis if the patient does not have access to a breast care center.

The General Assembly of the Commonwealth of Pennsylvania hereby enacts as follows:

Section 1. Short title.

This act shall be known and may be cited as the *Breast Care Center Treatment Act.*

Section 2. Legislation findings.

The General Assembly finds and declares as follows:

(1) Breast cancer is the most commonly diagnosed cancer among women in this Nation and in this Commonwealth. It is also the second leading cause of death in this Commonwealth.

(2) The Centers for Disease Control and Prevention have estimated that in 2005, 11,340 new cases of breast cancer will be diagnosed in Pennsylvania. The Department of Health estimates that approximately 2,300 women will have died of this disease in 2004.

(3) Studies have shown that the five-year survival rate for breast cancer is 96% if it is detected early. If detected in later stages, the survival rate declines to 21%.

(4) Studies have also shown 40% of general radiologists have missed breast cancer in their interpretations and readings of diagnostic tests.

(5) Leaders in the field of breast care have also stated that specialization in this disease results in better clinical outcomes and faster diagnosis. They have also stated: "Once a breast abnormality has been identified, no matter which health care provider identifies it, a referral to a breast care center should be the next step, and that referral should be for diagnostic evaluation in breast imaging. The radiologist, specialized in breast imaging, should then have the authority to refer the patient for treatment, based on the diagnosis that is made.

I'm also working at the federal level, and many breast cancer coalitions across the country are helping me. Once we harness our energy we can go to our congressmen and women and push hard to put a similar bill through at the federal level. This is a national campaign to end misdiagnosis, to make sure it doesn't happen to another woman in this country.

I still cry sometimes, not for the loss of my wife, but for the women who are living the same story or will be misdiagnosed like Maureen, losing their chance for early diagnosis, their right to be cured. Thank you for reading Maureen's story. I pray that this will never happen to you. That's why I will continue telling her story every chance I get. I pray for all the women in this country that a pamphlet will be handed to you, if you find a lump, with the guidelines of diagnosis, treatment and follow-up of your breast lump. Then you will be assured of an early diagnosis and most likely a correct one. I also pray that my bill The Breast Care Center Treatment Act will make it into law, for your safety. The promise I made to Maureen is now a promise I intend to keep for all the women in this country. I will do my best to ensure women an early, correct diagnosis.

Maureen Thiel died of breast cancer on May 16, 1998. After visits to three different doctors, from November 1994 to May of 1996, including a surgeon, and after multiple mammograms and ultrasounds, she was told, three different times, "Do not worry Mrs. Thiel, you have common cysts, come back in a year for your annual mammogram." Because she was never fully informed, never given an educational pamphlet on breast care, never told how to take charge of her own medical care, she relied on doctors, trusting them to diagnose her properly.

Maureen's story is a lesson for us all. None of Maureen's doctors were specialized in breast care. None of her doctors followed up on Maureen according to the standards in the guidelines of breast care. She did not know this. I know it now, and that is why Maureen made me promise to tell her story and save another woman's life. Her last wish was for me to let women know where to get the resources to educate themselves, so they wouldn't die as she did without a chance.

While it is very important to have early detection, it is just as important to have a correct diagnosis. Maureen's lump was detected in November 1994, but never correctly diagnosed until March of 1997. After her surgery, 47 out of 47 lymph nodes were positive and she was diagnosed with Stage III cancer. Her prognosis was less than two years of survival; she only lived 15 months. This didn't have to happen.

If you find a lump or a change in your breast and it is found to be abnormal, use the information in this book to make sure you receive the proper standard of care. Don't settle for anything less.

Bill Thiel, Executive Director: Maureen's Mission www.maureensmission.org

978-0-595-40747-7
0-595-40747-1